Blueprints Q&A
STEP 3: OBSTETRICS AND GYNECOLOGY

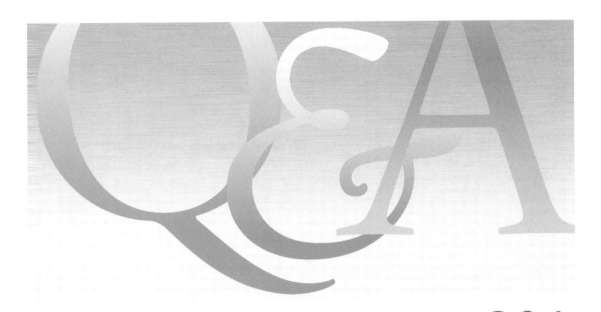

Blueprints Q&A
STEP 3: OBSTETRICS AND GYNECOLOGY

SERIES EDITOR:
Michael S. Clement, MD

AUTHORS:
Aaron B. Caughey, MD, MPP, MPH

Deirdre J. Lyell, MD

Susan H. Tran, MD

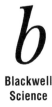

**Blackwell
Science**

EDITORIAL OFFICES:

Commerce Place, 350 Main Street,
  Malden, Massachusetts 02148, USA

Osney Mead, Oxford OX2 0EL, England

25 John Street, London WC1N 2BS, England

23 Ainslie Place, Edinburgh EH3 6AJ, Scotland

54 University Street, Carlton, Victoria 3053, Australia

OTHER EDITORIAL OFFICES:

Blackwell Wissenschafts-Verlag GmbH,
  Kurfürstendamm 57, 10707 Berlin, Germany

Blackwell Science KK, MG Kodenmacho Building,
  7-10 Kodenmacho Nihombashi, Chuo-ku,
  Tokyo 104, Japan

Iowa State University Press, A Blackwell Science Company,
  2121 S. State Avenue, Ames, Iowa 50014-8300, USA

DISTRIBUTORS:

The Americas
  Blackwell Publishing
  c/o AIDC
  P.O. Box 20
  50 Winter Sport Lane
  Williston, VT 05495-0020
  (Telephone orders: 800-216-2522;
  fax orders: 802-864-7626)

Australia Blackwell Science Pty, Ltd.
  54 University Street
  Carlton, Victoria 3053
  (Telephone orders: 03-9347-0300;
  fax orders: 03-9349-3016)

Outside The Americas and Australia
  Blackwell Science, Ltd.
  c/o Marston Book Services, Ltd., P.O. Box 269
  Abingdon, Oxon OX14 4YN, England
  (Telephone orders: 44-01235-465500;
  fax orders: 44-01235-465555)

Acquisitions: Beverly Copland

Development: Julia Casson

Production: Elissa Gershowitz

Manufacturing: Lisa Flanagan

Marketing Manager: Toni Fournier

Cover design by Hannus Design

Typeset by International Typesetting and Composition

Printed and bound by Courier-Stoughton

Printed in the United States of America

01 02 03 04 5 4 3 2 1

The Blackwell Science logo is a trade mark of Blackwell Science Ltd., registered at the United Kingdom Trade Marks Registry

Library of Congress Cataloging-in-Publication Data

Caughey, Aaron B.
Blueprints Q&A step 3. Obstetrics & gynecology /
by Aaron B. Caughey, Deirdre J. Lyell, Susan H. Tran.
     p. ; cm.—(Blueprints Q & A step 3 series)
  ISBN 0-632-04606-6 (pbk.)
  1. Obstetrics—Examinations, questions, etc.
  2. Gynecology—Examinations, questions, etc.
  3. Physicians—Licenses—United States—Examinations—
Study guides.
  [DNLM: 1. Genital Diseases, Female—Examination
Questions. 2. Delivery—Examination Questions.
3. Pregnancy Complications—Examination Questions.
WP 18.2 C371b 2002] I. Title: Blueprints Q and A step 3.
Obstetrics & gynecology. II. Title: Obstetrics &
gynecology. III. Lyell, Deirdre J. IV. Tran, Susan H. V. Title.
VI. Series.
  RG111 .C38 2002
    618'.076—dc21   2001006804

Notice: The indications and dosages of all drugs in this book have been recommended in the medical literature and conform to the practices of the general community. The medications described and treatment prescriptions suggested do not necessarily have specific approval by the Food and Drug Administration for use in the diseases and dosages for which they are recommended. The package insert for each drug should be consulted for use and dosage as approved by the FDA. Because standards for usage change, it is advisable to keep abreast of revised recommendations, particularly those concerning new drugs.

AUTHORS

Aaron B. Caughey, MD, MPP, MPH

Postdoctoral Fellow in the Department of Obstetrics
& Gynecology

University of California, San Francisco

Fellow in Maternal-Fetal Medicine

UCSF Medical Center/San Francisco General Hospital

Doctoral Candidate-Health Services and Policy
Analysis

University of California, Berkeley

San Francisco and Berkeley, California

Deirdre J. Lyell, MD

Clinical Instructor in Obstetrics and Gynecology

Stanford Medical School

Fellow in Maternal-Fetal Medicine

Department of Obstetrics and Gynecology

Stanford Medical Center

Stanford, California

Susan H. Tran, MD

Resident in Obstetrics and Gynecology

Department of Obstetrics and Gynecology

Kaiser Hospital, San Francisco

San Francisco, California

REVIEWERS

Mila Felder
Class of 2002
Chicago Medical School

Michelle Rorie, MD
Chief Resident
Department of Family and Community Medicine
Meharry Medical College

PREFACE

The Blueprints Q&A Step 3 series has been developed to complement our core content Blueprints books. Each Blueprints Q&A Step 3 book (*Medicine, Pediatrics, Surgery, Psychiatry,* and *Obstetrics/ Gynecology*) was written by residents seeking to provide the highest quality of practice review questions simulating the USMLE.

Like the actual USMLE Step 3 exam, this book is divided into different practice settings: Community-Based Health Center, Office, In-Patient Facility, and Emergency Department. Each book covers a single discipline, allowing you to use them during "down-time." Each book contains 100 review cases that cover content typical to the Step 3 USMLE.

Answers are found at the end of each setting, with the correct option highlighted. Accompanying the correct answer is a discussion of why the other options are incorrect. This allows for even the wrong answers to provide you with a valuable learning experience.

Blackwell has been fortunate to work with expert editors and residents—people like you who have studied for and passed the Boards. They sought to provide you with the very best practice prior to taking the Boards.

We welcome feedback and suggestions you may have about this book or any in the Blueprints series. Send to blue@blacksci.com.

All of the authors and staff at Blackwell wish you well on the Boards, and in your medical future!

ACKNOWLEDGMENTS

We all would like to thank the staff at Blackwell Science particularly Julia Casson and Bev Copland for involving us in this project. I would also like to thank my family, friends, and colleagues including the residents and faculty in the Departments of Obstetrics and Gynecology at UCSF and the Brigham and Women's Hospital, Dr. Peter Callen, the students, staff, and faculty at UC Berkeley's Health Services and Policy Analysis program and the Department of Economics, and as always my mother, father, Ethan, Samara, Big & Mugsy, D & Max, all of the new babies and fetuses (Nicole, Jacob, Kailee, Maia, Remy, baby Friel, and baby Mitchell) and of course, Bugsy whose unflagging support during all of my projects keeps me on task and productive.

Aaron B. Caughey, MD, MPP, MPH

This project is dedicated to the medical students, residents, faculty, and staff at Stanford Medical Center and the Brigham and Women's Hospital, my parents and siblings, and most of all to Jacob and Max.

Deirdre J. Lyell, MD

FIGURE CREDITS

Figure 8. Cox FEG. Modern Parasitology: A Textbook of Parasitology. 2nd ed. Oxford: Blackwell Science, 1993:9.

Figure 32A. Callahan TL, Caughey AB, Heffner LJ. Blueprints in Obstetrics and Gynecology. 2nd ed. Malden, MA: Blackwell Science, 2001:98

Figure 32B. Callahan TL, Caughey AB, Heffner LJ. Blueprints in Obstetrics and Gynecology. 2nd ed. Malden, MA: Blackwell Science, 2001:99

Figure 42. Visual Graphics, Inc. of Boca Raton, Florida.

Figure 45. Crissey JT. Manual of Medical Mycology. Malden: Blackwell Science, 1995:90.

Figure 50. Visual Graphics, Inc. of Boca Raton, Florida.

Figure 51A. Visual Graphics, Inc. of Boca Raton, Florida.

Figure 51B. Visual Graphics, Inc. of Boca Raton, Florida.

Figure 56. Visual Graphics, Inc. of Boca Raton, Florida.

Figure 63. Creasy R. Management of Labor and Delivery, Malden: Blackwell Science, 1997.

Figure 89. Visual Graphics, Inc. of Boca Raton, Florida.

Figure 90. Clark SL, et al. Critical Care Obstetrics. 2nd ed. Cambridge: Blackwell Science, 1991:163.

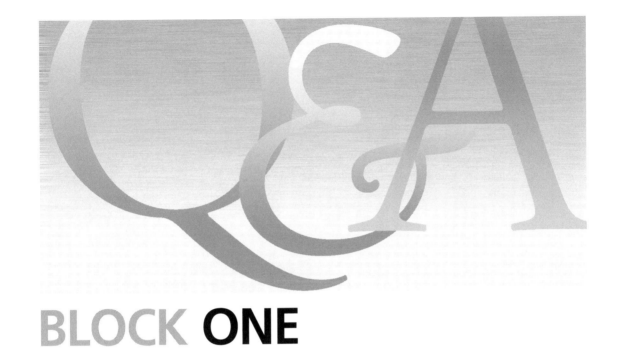

BLOCK **ONE**

QUESTIONS

Setting I: Community-Based Health Center

This is a community-based health facility where patients seeking both routine and urgent care are encountered. Many patients are low income; many are ethnic minorities. Several industrial parks and local small businesses send employees there with on-the-job injuries and for employee health screening. There is facility for x-ray films, but CT and MRI must be arranged at other facilities. Laboratory services are available.

QUESTION 1

A 23-year-old G1P0 presents for a routine office visit at 24 weeks gestational age (GA). Her pregnancy has been remarkable for nausea and vomiting early on that has resolved. She is generally healthy and has had a single urinary tract infection in her life. She denies dysuria, fevers, chills, contractions, vaginal bleeding, and leakage of fluid, and reports good fetal movement. Her blood pressure is 90/60. A routine urine dipstick in clinic reveals 1+ protein, trace blood, trace leukocyte esterase, and 1+ white blood cells. The most appropriate next step is:

A. Send a urine culture.

B. Counsel her to follow up if she becomes symptomatic.

C. Treat with antibiotics.

D. Do nothing.

E. Renal biopsy.

QUESTION 2

A mother brings her 16-year-old G0 daughter to clinic, concerned because the daughter has not yet begun to menstruate. On exam, the patient is 5 ft 9 in. tall and weighs 120 lb. Her breasts are elevated and enlarged, and the areolae project to form a secondary mound. She shaves her axilla and has mid-escutcheon on her mons. Her vagina appears well estrogenized, there is no septum seen, and her cervix appears normal. On palpation, a uterus is present, and her ovaries feel normal. Which Tanner stage of development best describes this patient?

A. Stage 1

B. Stage 2

C. Stage 3

D. Stage 4

E. Stage 5

QUESTION 3

A 16-year-old G0 Caucasian female is brought in by her mother for what appears to be primary amenorrhea. However, upon further questioning she admits that she had her first period at age 14, had four periods every 1–2 months after that, and has not had a period for more than 7 months. She denies abdominal pain but reports her periods were previously painful. When questioned alone, the patient reports that she is sexually active with her boyfriend of 1 year with rare condom usage. She had a Pap smear and testing for gonorrhea and chlamydia 5 months ago at a neighborhood teen clinic, both of which she reports were normal. She considered taking oral contraceptive pills in the past but states that she does not want to gain weight from the pills. She has no medical problems and has never had surgery. She is 5 ft 7 in. tall and weighs 100 lb. Her exam is normal and development is otherwise appropriate for her age. A urine pregnancy test is negative. What is the most likely cause of this patient's secondary amenorrhea?

A. Cervical stenosis

B. Asherman's syndrome

C. Premature ovarian failure

D. Hypothalamic

E. Polycystic ovarian disease

QUESTION 4

A 32-year-old G0 presents to clinic for a preconceptional visit. In addition to testing for rubella immunity, inquiring about a history of chicken pox, prescribing prenatal vitamins, and discussing the optimal mid-cycle timing for conception, you ask if she drinks alcohol, uses recreational drugs, or smokes cigarettes. She says that she never drinks alcohol or uses recreational drugs, but does smoke two packs of cigarettes each day. All of the following are true EXCEPT:

A. Infants of women who smoked during pregnancy are at increased risk of sudden infant death syndrome (SIDS) and respiratory illnesses in childhood.

B. Approximately 40% of women who are smokers at the time of conception are able to quit by the time of their first prenatal visit.

C. Smoking more than one pack per day is more harmful than smoking less than one pack per day.

D. Smoking during pregnancy is associated with spontaneous abortion, abruption, and decreased birth weight.

E. Smoking cessation is more effective during pregnancy.

QUESTION 5

A 32-year-old G4P3-0-0-3 (term deliveries/preterm deliveries/abortions/live children) sees you for her second prenatal visit at 15 weeks GA. She had agreed to a human immunodeficiency virus (HIV) test at her first visit, which is part of the universal screening that your clinic offers. Both the Western Blot and Elisa are positive for HIV. The patient has never received a blood transfusion or used intravenous drugs. She works as a maid in a hotel where she cleans rooms and has no known work-related exposures. She is monogamous with her husband and believes their relationship to be mutually monogamous. He has no known exposures. She feels well in general and has had no symptoms of opportunistic infections. You counsel her all of the following EXCEPT:

A. The patient's husband should be tested for HIV.

B. There is no known cure for HIV.

C. Without antiretroviral prophylaxis, approximately 25% of infants born to HIV infected women will become infected with HIV.

D. Immunoglobulins from breast-feeding may protect the infant from HIV infection.

E. Increased vertical transmission is seen among patients with higher viral loads and more advanced disease.

QUESTION 6

A 24-year-old G1P1 African American woman presents for her 6-week postpartum visit. She had presented in preterm labor at $34^6/_7$ weeks GA and delivered 24 hrs later at 35 weeks. Her daughter spent 1 week in the neonatal intensive care unit, but has done well since discharge. The patient's prenatal care had been entirely uncomplicated until delivery. She had presented to you for her first prenatal visit at 9 weeks GA, and all the labs in the first and second trimesters were normal. All of the following are true EXCEPT:

A. Perinatal morbidity is higher among African Americans when compared to Caucasians.

B. Perinatal mortality among African Americans is higher than in Caucasians.

C. Premature African American infants have a higher rate of respiratory distress syndrome compared to GA-matched Caucasian infants.

D. On average, African American patients present for prenatal care at a greater GA than Caucasians.

E. African Americans have a higher incidence of preterm delivery when compared to Caucasians.

QUESTION 7

A 19-year-old G1P0 woman presents at 29 weeks GA complaining of constant abdominal pain for 2 days and leakage of fluid for approximately 1 week. She feels otherwise well and denies fevers, chills, nausea, vomiting, diarrhea, and dysuria. Her appetite is normal. On exam, she is febrile to 102.2°F (39°C), her pulse is 120, her uterus is tender to palpation, and she has a foul-smelling, purulent vaginal discharge. There is no pool of fluid in her vagina, but a fluid sample is positive for both ferning and nitrazine. The patient's cervix appears long and closed. Office ultrasound reveals a cephalic presentation, an amniotic fluid index of 2, and a fetal heart rate in the 170s. You transfer her to labor and delivery. The most appropriate next step is:

A. Cesarean section

B. Antibiotics and observation

C. Amniocentesis for culture

D. Tampon dye test

E. Induction of labor

QUESTION 8

A 21-year-old G0 presents complaining of profuse, foul-smelling greenish vaginal discharge. Her symptoms worsened 2 days after the end of her last menstrual period. She also complains of itching and irritation. She is sexually active, has had two partners in the last 3 months, and does not use condoms. On sterile speculum, she has a frothy gray-green discharge. You perform a wet prep in clinic and see actively moving, flagellated organisms on wet prep. Which of the following is true regarding this patient? See Figure 8.

A. She can be treated with 2 g of oral metronidazole (Flagyl).

B. Her partners do not need treatment, as this is not a sexually transmitted disease.

C. She can be treated with 250 mg of oral azithromycin (Zithromax).

D. Since this is not a sexually transmitted disease, she does not need to be screened for sexually transmitted diseases.

E. Prior to treatment, a culture should be sent to confirm diagnosis, which cannot be made on wet prep alone.

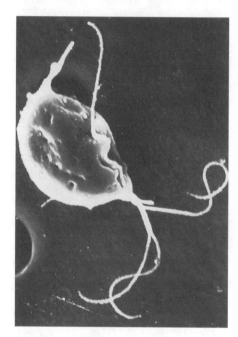

FIGURE 8

QUESTION 9

An 18-year-old G1P0 presents at 21 weeks GA complaining of a persistent trickle of fluid that began 3 hr ago. She denies contractions, vaginal bleeding, fever, chills, abnormal discharge, dysuria, or abdominal pain. She reports an unsure LMP (last menstrual period) and was dated by an 18-week ultrasound that was consistent with a $15^5/_7$ weeks GA fetus. There were no anomalies identified on ultrasound. The patient smokes two packs of cigarettes per day. Physical exam is within normal limits. However, sterile speculum exam confirms a pool of fluid that turns nitrazine paper deep blue and crystallizes on a slide causing a fern pattern. Which of the following would be INAPPROPRIATE in the management of this patient?

A. Expectant management at home

B. Dilation and evacuation

C. Cervical cerclage

D. Ultrasound

E. Observation on labor and delivery

QUESTION 10

A 31-year-old G4P3 woman presents to clinic at 33 weeks GA complaining of feeling like she wets herself constantly. She describes having felt increased wetness for approximately 4 weeks. She has no medical problems, and her pregnancy has been uncomplicated. She experiences occasional vaginal itching and mild pain. She denies contractions, vaginal bleeding, abnormal discharge, and reports active fetal movement. What is the most appropriate next step in this patient's management?

A. Observation at home with further evaluation if the symptoms worsen

B. Sterile speculum exam with tests for ferning and nitrazine

C. Sterile speculum exam with a KOH and wet prep

D. Swab for Group B streptococcus

E. Ultrasound

QUESTION 11

A 22-year-old G0 woman complains of a foul-smelling vaginal discharge and dyspareunia for 3 days. She has been sexually active with her new partner for 1 month and uses oral contraception, but not condoms. She has had two other sexual partners during the last year, and did not use condoms with either. Her last menstrual period was 8 days ago. She is compliant and well known to you. On exam, she is afebrile and her abdomen is nontender. Her pelvic exam is significant for scant vaginal discharge, mucopurulent discharge coming from her cervical os, cervical-motion tenderness, and nontender uterus and adnexa. Treatment includes all of the following EXCEPT:

A. Ceftriaxone 250 mg IM once and doxycycline 100 mg po bid for 14 days

B. Cefoxitin 2 g IV q6 hr and doxycycline 100 mg IV q12 hr until afebrile for 48 hr

C. Ofloxacillin 400 mg po once and azithromycin 1 g po once

D. Azithromycin 2 g po once

E. Ceftriaxone 250 mg IM once and azithromycin 1 g po once

QUESTION 12

A 27-year-old G0 woman and her boyfriend present for contraceptive advice. For the past 2 months they have used periodic abstinence (the rhythm method) for birth control. Which of the following is FALSE regarding actual contraceptive failure rates within the first year of use of each method?

A. Condom: 12%

B. No method: 85%

C. Copper T intrauterine device (IUD): 0.7%

D. Vasectomy: 0.15%

E. Combination oral contraceptive pill: 0.5%

QUESTION 13

A 32-year-old G4P0-1-2-0 presents for her first prenatal visit at 31 weeks GA. She is homeless, and her pregnancy was discovered when she presented for amenorrhea to the Mobile Medical Outreach Clinic, which visits her area weekly. She is concerned because she uses heroin daily, and has done so for the past 4 months. She denies other drug or alcohol use. She has been intermittently homeless for several years. She occasionally lives with a male friend. She is otherwise healthy. You recommend that she does all of the following today EXCEPT:

A. Stop all narcotics.

B. Undergo all of the first trimester labs.

C. Begin methadone.

D. Undergo ultrasound.

E. Test for HIV.

QUESTION 14

A 29-year-old G2P1-0-0-1 at 39 weeks GA calls your office concerned because her nephew, who spent the day with her yesterday, has just been diagnosed with chicken pox. The patient does not recall a history of chicken pox. She is feeling well and has no medical problems. She denies fever, chills, or a rash. Her pregnancy has been uncomplicated. You recommend that she does which of the following:

A. Go to clinic for an exam.

B. Go to the emergency department for varicella-zoster immune globulin (VZIG).

C. Go to the pharmacy and fill a prescription for oral acyclovir.

D. Alert the pediatrician so that the infant may be prophylaxed after delivery.

E. Go to the emergency department for a VZV titer.

QUESTION 15

A 27-year-old Asian woman presents for her annual exam. She was diagnosed with HIV one year ago and has not received gynecologic care since. Six years ago she was treated for low-grade squamous intraepithelial neoplasia (LGSIL). She had frequent follow-up with colposcopy and Pap smear, all of which were negative. She was eventually discharged to routine care. You plan to perform a Pap smear today. All of the following are true EXCEPT:

A. The patient should have repeat Pap smears every 6 months.

B. Cervical cancer is considered an AIDS defining illness in HIV-positive women.

C. Otherwise healthy HIV-infected women without symptomatic HIV or previous abnormal Pap smears may undergo Pap smears annually.

D. The incidence of invasive cervical cancer is similar to that of non-HIV-infected women.

E. Human papilloma virus (HPV) and HIV act synergistically and cause cervical cancer.

QUESTION 16

A 48-year-old G2P2 African American woman presents with menorrhagia. She also complains of bloating and pelvic pressure. She notes that during the past 2 years her menses have become longer and heavier. She has also begun to experience dyspareunia and constipation. Fullness is palpated on rectovaginal exam. A pelvic ultrasound reveals an $8 \times 8 \times 6$ cm homogenous fibroid in the posterior uterine wall. Which of the following is true about fibroids? See Figure 16.

A. Most women with fibroids eventually become symptomatic.

B. Fibroids should be removed because of their malignant potential.

C. Fibroids tend to regress during pregnancy.

D. Fibroids are associated with infertility.

E. Fibroids are most common among Latino women.

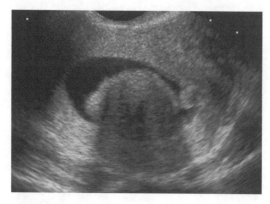

FIGURE 16

QUESTION 17

A 23-year-old G2P0 Asian woman presents to your office at 13 weeks GA after receiving notification that an RPR test performed during her first prenatal visit last week was reactive. She denies arthritis, fever, rash, and photosensitivity, but reports worsening intermittent fatigue during the last 2 years, which is not significant enough to prevent her from exercising. She has no medical problems, and takes no medications. She has had three sexual partners during the last year, and notes sexual contact with two of the partners in the last 3 months with only occasional use of condoms. She had a full STD screen 1 year ago, including an RPR, which was negative. The most appropriate next step is:

A. Send an ANA.

B. Arrange a consult with rheumatology.

C. Send an MHA-TP.

D. Treat with benzathine penicillin G.

E. Repeat the RPR.

QUESTION 18

A 31-year-old G3P3 Latino woman is found to have CIN III on her Pap smear. Colposcopically directed biopsies are consistent with CIN III at two sites on the exocervix, as well as on a lesion that appears to extend into the endocervix. The endocervical curettage is normal. The patient has always had normal annual Pap smears, with the most recent being 1 year ago. She has had a new sexual partner for the last 6 months, and uses oral contraception. The most appropriate next step in treatment is:

A. Serotype for HPV

B. Cryotherapy

C. Laser ablation of the lesion

D. Loop electrosurgical excision procedure (LEEP) or cold knife cone (CKC)

E. Repeat colposcopy and biopsies in 3 months

QUESTION 19

A 19-year-old presents to clinic complaining of amenorrhea and breast tenderness for 2 months. A urine pregnancy test is positive. She has been using a diaphragm with spermicide for contraception. She was counseled regarding proper diaphragm use when her diaphragm was fit 1 year ago. Which of the following is FALSE regarding optimal diaphragm use?

A. The diaphragm should be removed 2–3 hr after intercourse.

B. If a couple has intercourse again prior to diaphragm removal, additional spermicide should be used.

C. The diaphragm should be replaced every 5 years.

D. The diaphragm can cause toxic shock syndrome if left in place for too long.

E. The actual annual failure rate of the diaphragm is greater than 10%.

QUESTION 20

A 38-year-old G0 African American pre-menopausal woman presents to clinic for an annual exam. Her last exam was 3 years ago. She is 5 ft 7 in. tall and weighs 129 lb. Her physical exam is within normal limits except for the pelvic exam. On bimanual exam, you note a left adnexal mass, distinct from her uterus, which is retroverted and retroflexed. The mass is non-tender and palpates approximately 6–7 cm in diameter. You order a pelvic ultrasound, which reveals an 8 × 7 × 5 cm complex left ovarian mass. There is no ascites or omental thickening seen. The other ovary appears entirely normal. When considering how to counsel this patient about her differential diagnosis, which of the following is FALSE regarding types of major ovarian tumors?

A. Germ cell tumors include mucinous and endometrioid tumors.

B. Epithelial cell tumors are the most common.

C. Sex-cord stromal tumors include granulosa-theca and Sertoli-Leydig tumors.

D. Epithelial cell tumors are more frequent among women in their late 50s.

E. Germ cell tumors are more frequent among girls and young women.

QUESTION 21

A 37-year-old G2P1-0-0-1 Caucasian woman well known to you from her first pregnancy presents to you at 33 weeks GA with her third complaint of decreased fetal movement in the last 3 weeks. You send her for a non-stress test, which is reactive, and she appears tremendously relieved. She had an amniocentesis at 16 weeks GA that was normal and an obstetric ultrasound at 20 weeks GA that revealed an appropriately grown fetus without identifiable anomalies and a posterior placenta. Her fundal height measures appropriately. She is 5 ft 5 in. and has gained only 8 lb during this pregnancy. She reports that she has had difficulty eating well because of poor appetite, but has been trying to increase her caloric intake. She is married and describes her husband as somewhat ambivalent about the pregnancy because of financial concerns. During this pregnancy, she has come in almost weekly complaining of numerous nonspecific symptoms, including headache, abdominal pain, decreased fetal movement, joint pain, and heartburn. You recall that she did not have these multiple somatic complaints during her first pregnancy. The most important next step in management is:

A. Biophysical profile

B. Detailed history and physical with emphasis on social history

C. Screening for anorexia nervosa

D. Ultrasound

E. Weekly non-stress tests (NST)

QUESTION 22

A 23-year-old G3P0 Caucasian woman presents at 25 weeks GA for a prenatal appointment. She has not been seen since her first prenatal appointment at 12 weeks GA. She has a history of polysubstance abuse and two second-trimester abortions. She is 5 ft 5 in. tall and weighs 107 lb. Her blood pressure is 149/88. You are unable to obtain fetal heart tones and perform an ultrasound, which confirms that the fetus has no heart activity. On further ultrasound examination, you note a large retroplacental clot and fetal biometry consistent with 22 weeks GA. The patient is quite upset by these findings, but after she has a chance to calm down and call her sister, you obtain further history that she has been using her drug of choice pretty heavily over the past 2 months. She also notes that she has had some vaginal bleeding for the past 3 weeks. Which of the following is most likely to be found on urine tox screen?

A. Marijuana

B. Ethanol

C. Benzodiazepines

D. Cocaine

E. Heroin (opiates)

QUESTION 23

A mother brings her 15-year-old daughter to clinic, concerned because of her daughter's abdominal pain. The pain began 2 months prior and has become constant. She is virginal and in good health. She has normal monthly menses and denies fevers, chills, nausea, vomiting, and weight loss. Pelvic ultrasound reveals a complex 8×6 cm left ovarian mass. Which of the following is FALSE regarding the association between germ cell tumors and serum tumor markers?

A. Choriocarcinoma and human chorionic gonadotropin (hCG)

B. Dysgerminoma and alpha-fetoprotein (AFP)

C. Embryonal carcinoma and hCG, and AFP

D. Endodermal sinus tumor and AFP

E. Immature teratoma and CA-125

QUESTION 24

A 62-year-old G2P2 woman, menopausal for 12 years, presents to clinic complaining of abdominal bloating for 6 months. During the past 2 months she has been unable to button her pants, despite a 10-lb weight loss achieved without dieting. A pelvic ultrasound reveals massive ascites and a 9 × 10 cm complex right ovarian mass. In addition to obtaining lab work, the next step in management is:

A. Observation with repeat ultrasound in 4 weeks

B. Exploratory laparotomy

C. Diuretic treatment for relief of her ascites

D. A second opinion

E. Chemotherapy

QUESTION 25

A 26-year-old G0 Caucasian woman presents complaining that she hasn't had a period for 3 months. She began menstruating at the age of 12 and had fairly regular cycles, every 28–30 days, until they became somewhat irregular 2 years ago. She describes cycle lengths of 35–37 days, with occasional months when she misses her period altogether. Some months, her period is moderate to heavy, lasting 5–7 days, and other months it lasts only 1–2 days and is quite light. She has no medical problems. Since the death of her mother 3 years ago, she has gained approximately 40 lb. She admits that she eats in response to stress, and is seeking counseling for this. She is not currently sexually active. She last had intercourse 4 months ago, and used a condom for contraception. On exam, she is 5 ft 4 in. tall and weighs 180 lb. Her skin is clear. She is hirsute on her upper lip, chin, and forearms. Her lung, cardiac, and breast exams are normal. Her abdomen is soft, nontender, and without palpable masses. Her uterus is difficult to palpate, as are her adnexa. What is the most important first test to order in this patient?

A. Serum testosterone level

B. TSH

C. Prolactin

D. Glucose tolerance test

E. Urine HCG

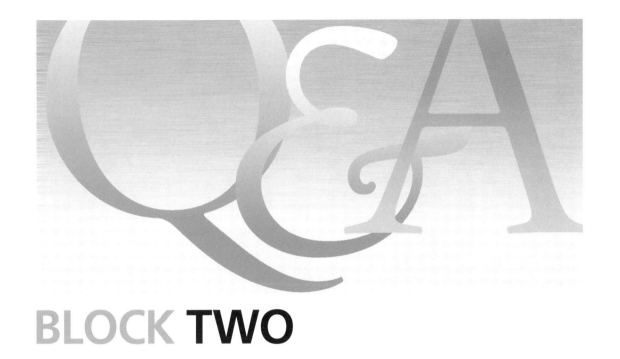

BLOCK **TWO**

QUESTIONS

Setting II: Office

Your office is in a primary care generalist group practice located in a physician office suite adjoining a suburban community hospital. Patients are usually seen by appointment. Most of the patients you see are from your own practice and are appearing for regular scheduled return visits, with some new patients. As in most group practices, you will encounter a patient whose primary care is managed by one of your associates; reference may be made to the patient's medical records. You may do some telephone management and you may have to respond to questions about articles in magazines and on TV that will require interpretation. The laboratory and radiology services are complete.

QUESTION 26

A 26-year-old G2P0 woman presents for her first prenatal appointment. She is generally healthy, with seasonal allergies and no history of prior surgeries. She reports that her menstrual periods come every month, and the last one was about 5 months ago. When you ask her to be more specific about the day, she can only answer that it was between the first and the ninth days of that month. You order an ultrasound to help with the dating of the pregnancy. Which of the following is the best method to date a pregnancy when used alone?

A. Last menstrual period (LMP)

B. First trimester ultrasound

C. Second trimester ultrasound

D. Third trimester ultrasound

E. Quantitative beta-HCG correlated with dates

QUESTION 27

A 17-year-old G1P0 Caucasian woman presents to your office. She is sexually active in a monogamous relationship and has been using condoms for contraception. She is concerned because she has not had her period for 6 weeks and wonders if she might be pregnant. Her medical history is unremarkable and she is currently in her senior year of high school. On review of systems, she does note some mild nausea over the past week that comes and goes throughout the day, as well as increasing breast tenderness, which she thought meant her period was due at any moment. She has had no spotting or pelvic pain. Her urine pregnancy test is positive for pregnancy, and her physical exam is consistent with an early first trimester intrauterine gestation. She asks you about nonsurgical options for termination of pregnancy. You tell her that all of the following medical interventions have been used for termination of pregnancy in the first trimester EXCEPT:

A. Mifepristone (RU-486)

B. Misoprostol (Cytotec) alone

C. Misoprostol plus methotrexate

D. Misoprostol plus mifepristone

E. High dose estrogen/progesterone pills given every 12 hr

QUESTION 28

A couple presents to your office with complaints of infertility. He is 38 and she is 39. They have been trying to get pregnant for 9 months by attempting to time intercourse with her ovulation. However, her periods are irregular and it has been difficult to determine when ovulation is occurring. His semen analysis returns within normal limits. You suggest testing her for ovulation, which can be performed by all of the following EXCEPT:

A. An LH/FSH ratio

B. Basal body temperature testing

C. A progesterone level in the mid-luteal phase

D. Urine LH measurement

E. Endometrial biopsy

QUESTION 29

A 24-year-old G1P0 woman at $10^3/_7$ weeks GA presents for prenatal care. She has no prior medical history, had an appendectomy at age 11, and has no family history of diabetes. Her initial physical exam is entirely within normal limits and consistent with her dating. In addition to this initial history and physical, you send her for prenatal labs. Which of the following is UNNECESSARY at this point?

A. RPR

B. Rubella titer

C. Hepatitis B surface antigen

D. MSAFP (maternal serum alpha fetoprotein)

E. CBC

QUESTION 30

A 36-year-old G2P1 Asian woman presents for her fourth prenatal visit at 17 weeks GA. She had some nausea and vomiting in the first trimester that resolved by 14 weeks GA and otherwise has had an entirely uncomplicated pregnancy. At her last appointment at 15 weeks GA, she underwent screening for maternal serum alpha-fetoprotein (MSAFP). The result returned 2 days ago with a value that is 4.5 multiples of the median (MoMs). Which of the following would NOT be an etiology of this abnormal result?

A. Anencephaly

B. Twin gestation

C. Gastroschisis

D. Trisomy 18

E. She is actually 19 weeks gestational age

QUESTION 31

A 32-year-old G4P3 Latina presents for her 19-week prenatal care appointment immediately prior to her scheduled ultrasound. She has had an uncomplicated antenatal course with normal first trimester labs. In addition, her triple screen returned negative for neural tube defects or aneuploidy. She and her husband are looking forward to the ultrasound because they have three daughters and are hoping for a son. You tell her that which of the following is NOT a routine aspect of a Level I obstetric ultrasound:

A. Fetal extremities

B. Fetal number

C. Fetal kidneys

D. Amniotic fluid volume

E. Placental location

QUESTION 32

A 23-year-old G0 woman presents to your clinic with complaints of a tender mass near the left side of her vagina. She noticed the mass several weeks ago, but at that time it was only 1 cm in diameter and did not hurt. Over the past 3 days, however, the mass has increased in size and hurts continuously. The pain is mildly relieved by tub baths as well as the combination of acetaminophen and ibuprofen. She has been sexually active recently, but not over the past week because of discomfort. On physical exam, she has mild left inguinal lymphadenopathy. Her left external genitalia are swollen and focally erythematous around a 3–4-cm mass. See Figures 32A and 32B. Upon closer inspection, you note the mass is just inside the labia majora and outside of the hymeneal ring. It is quite tender to palpation and feels slightly fluctuant and tense. On rectal exam, there is no evidence of the mass impinging on the rectum and the patient denies rectal tenderness. You diagnose her with:

A. Vulvar abscess

B. Vaginal abscess

C. Herpes labialis

D. Bartholin's abscess

E. Condyloma

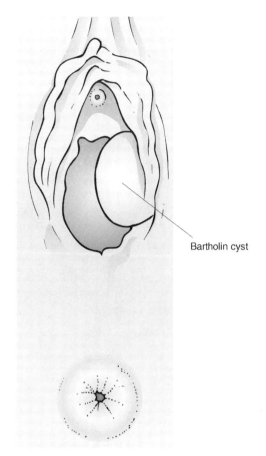

Bartholin cyst

FIGURE 32A

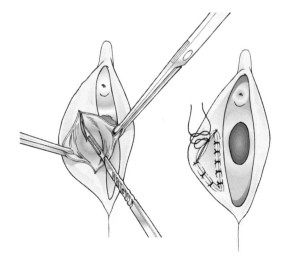

FIGURE 32B

QUESTION 33

A 37-year-old African American G1P0 woman at 41 weeks GA presents for her routine prenatal visit. Her pregnancy is complicated by a history of severe hyperemesis gravidarum until 16 weeks GA that required two brief hospital stays for aggressive hydration. She has felt fine for the second half of her pregnancy. All of her routine prenatal labs have been within normal limits, and she had an amniocentesis performed at 15 weeks, which revealed a 46, XX fetus. She now presents 1 week after her due date wanting to know when she will deliver. On examination, her cervix is closed but soft, and 50% effaced. You tell her that you will begin antenatal testing with a non-stress test. If it is reactive, you will reassure her that she is at lower risk for what condition over the ensuing week?

A. Gestational diabetes

B. Intrauterine fetal demise (IUFD)

C. Meconium in the amniotic fluid

D. Macrosomia

E. Preeclampsia

QUESTION 34

A 33-year-old G3P2 Caucasian patient at 14 weeks GA presents for her second prenatal visit. She had two prior uncomplicated births, a daughter, 7, and a son, 3. Her first trimester prenatal labs done at 11 weeks of gestation reveal that she is Rh negative and has an anti-D antibody titer of 1:4. She found out that she was Rh negative in her first pregnancy, and her daughter, at birth, was also Rh negative. Her last pregnancy was uncomplicated, and she had a negative antibody titer throughout. Her son was Rh positive. She received Rhogam (anti-D immune globulin) in her last two pregnancies at 28 weeks GA, but not after delivery in either one. Her Caucasian husband is the father of all of her pregnancies. Given that the rate of Rh negative individuals is 16% among Caucasians, which of the following is true about this patient?

(Reminder: The Hardy–Weinberg equation is $p^2 + 2pq + q^2 = 1$, where p = probability of dominant allele and q = probability of recessive allele)

A. Her husband has a 48% chance of being heterozygous.

B. There is a possibility that her husband is Rh negative.

C. The probability that this fetus is Rh negative is $pq/(2pq)$.

D. A dose of Rhogam in this pregnancy will be protective.

E. This patient will need serial amniocentesis in this pregnancy if the fetus is Rh positive.

QUESTION 35

A 49-year-old woman presents complaining of intermittent hot and cold spells, irregular periods, and mood swings. She notes these symptoms began 4 months ago and has been increasing in severity and frequency. On review of systems, she has no changes in diet, but does note that it is more difficult to sleep regularly. On physical exam, she has no breast lesions, a normal pelvic exam, and you send a Pap smear for evaluation. In addition, you order a TSH and FSH. The FSH returns elevated, while the TSH is normal. You offer the patient cyclic estrogen and progesterone, which will positively impact all of the following EXCEPT:

A. Her hot flashes

B. Her irregular periods

C. Osteoporosis

D. Cardiovascular disease

E. Her risk of stroke

QUESTION 36

A 13-year-old African American adolescent female presents to your office with complaints of lower abdominal pain that began 6 months ago. The pain lasts for 4–6 days and then decreases. For the last 2 months, the pain has lasted longer, and the patient now notes a fullness in her lower abdomen. She is not sexually active and has not begun menstruating yet. On physical exam she is Tanner stage III, and on abdominal exam you note mild lower abdominal tenderness and a palpable fullness in her lower abdomen. On pelvic exam you note that she has an intact hymeneal ring and a foreshortened vaginal vault of only 2 cm. Her most likely diagnosis is:

A. Testicular feminization

B. Imperforate hymen

C. Transverse vaginal septum

D. Labial fusion

E. Rudimentary uterine horn

QUESTION 37

A 27-year-old G3P2 woman presents to your office at 19 weeks GA after just having had her obstetric ultrasound. You call the ultrasonologist for the results and find that the fetus had a normal ultrasound except for a unilateral choroid plexus cyst in the right cerebral lateral ventricle. See Figure 37. Pregnancy has been uncomplicated to this point, and her second trimester serum screening results returned with lower than age-related risk of trisomies 21 and 18. You prepare to tell her that this finding has been associated with which of the following?

A. Trisomy 18

B. Anencephaly

C. Neural tube defects

D. Developmental delay

E. Turner's syndrome

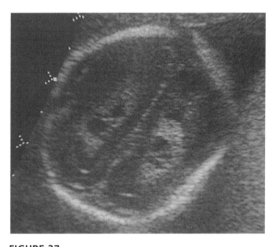

FIGURE 37

QUESTION 38

A 19-year-old G0 Caucasian woman presents to your office with complaints of lower abdominal and pelvic pain. She has had cyclic pain with her menses since the age of 14, but notes that over the past 12–15 months this pain has been increasing, leading to her inability to go to work for 2–3 days each month. For the past 2 months, she notes that she has pain that occurs several times between her periods and lasts for several days. She has been sexually active since age 15, has used only condoms for contraception, and has never had any pelvic infections to her knowledge. She is currently in a monogamous sexual relationship. However, she has not been sexually active for the past month secondary to dyspareunia. She does note some relief of symptoms with 400 mg of ibuprofen. The next step in her diagnosis and treatment is:

A. Laparoscopic resection of adhesions

B. Monophasic or continuous oral contraceptives

C. Gonadotropin releasing hormone (Lupron)

D. Pain consult/Psychiatry consult

E. Antibiotics

QUESTION 39

A 19-year-old G2P1 Latina woman presents to your office at 31 weeks GA. Her last visit was at 26 weeks GA, and she underwent her diabetes-screening test at that time which was normal. She has had no problems over the last 5 weeks and notes that she had rescheduled an appointment made 2 weeks prior because her 21-month-old daughter was sick. On physical exam, her fundal height measures 27 cm and a fetal heart rate is in the 140s. You review her records and see that her fundal height was 25 cm at the last visit and her daughter's birthweight was 3200 g. She weighs 67 kg and her birthweight was 2700 g. You obtain an ultrasound for fetal measurement because of size less than dates (S<D). Which of the following would NOT be an etiology of a fetus that is small for gestational age (SGA)?

A. Viral infections (e.g., cytomegalovirus)

B. Chromosomal abnormalities

C. Latina ethnicity

D. Chronic hypertension

E. Low maternal birthweight

QUESTION 40

A 29-year-old G2P1 woman presents at 27 weeks GA for a routine prenatal visit and third trimester labs. She has had an uncomplicated antenatal course up to this point. She weighs 82 kg now and her 3-year-old son's birthweight was 4300 g. She had a long labor with his delivery that resulted in a cesarean section when she had failed to dilate beyond 7 cm. She had an elevated glucose loading test (GLT) in her last pregnancy of 147, but a normal 3-hour glucose tolerance test (GTT) of 80, 177, 151, and 122. She has a maternal aunt who developed diabetes at age 57, but no other relatives with diabetes. You counsel her that in her history, which of the following is the biggest risk for her to have gestational diabetes in this pregnancy?

A. Previous elevated GLT

B. Prior macrosomic fetus

C. Aunt with type II diabetes

D. Her prior gestational diabetes

E. Her prior cesarean delivery

QUESTION 41

A 22-year-old G0 Korean woman presents with complaints of increased body and facial hair. She has noticed increased hair growth on her upper lip, chin, upper back, and lower abdomen for about 5 years. She denies deepening of her voice, balding, or enlargement of her clitoris. None of the other women in her family has any of these symptoms, and she feels quite self-conscious as a result. She underwent menarche at age 13, has irregular menses every 25–45 days, and has never been sexually active. On physical exam, she is 5 ft 4 in. tall and weighs 154 lb. She has some generalized acne on her face and back in addition to acanthosis nigricans. There are a few terminal hairs on her back as well as some stubble on her cheeks and upper lip. Her escutcheon is diamond-shaped. You send some lab tests which return with 17-α-hydroxyprogesterone, normal testosterone, a luteinizing hormone to follicle stimulating hormone ratio of 4, normal DHEA-S, and normal function of the 5-α-reductase. Her most likely diagnosis is:

A. Sertoli-Leydig cell tumor

B. Congenital adrenal hyperplasia

C. Testicular feminization

D. Germ cell tumor

E. Polycystic ovarian syndrome

QUESTION 42

A 76-year-old G7P4 woman presents with a complaint that something is falling out of her vagina. She notes that she started noticing a lump at her introitus while wiping several months ago, but it didn't bother her so she gave it no thought. Now she notes that occasionally this mass rubs between her labia while she is walking, which is uncomfortable. She underwent menopause at age 49 and has not taken HRT. She has mild COPD, a 60 pack per year history of smoking, and she still smokes one pack a day. On physical exam, her external exam reveals atrophic labia with fusion of the labia majora and minora. On speculum exam her vaginal mucosa is thin and atrophic as well. Her cervix is excoriated and on bimanual exam sits 1–2 cm inside the vaginal vault. When she stands, the cervix appears just between the labia and with cough extends beyond the labia approximately 1 cm. See Figure 42. Treatment of her third-degree uterine prolapse can involve all of the following EXCEPT:

A. Vaginal pessary

B. Estrogen cream

C. Kegel exercises

D. Burch culposuspension

E. Sacrospinous ligament suspension

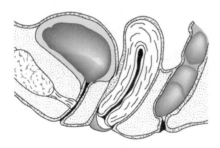

FIGURE 42

QUESTION 43

A 37-year-old G3P2 woman presents to your office at 12 weeks GA for her first prenatal visit. Her last two pregnancies were both complicated by late third-trimester preeclampsia, and after her second pregnancy she was diagnosed with hypertension and begun on antihypertensive medication. Prior to this pregnancy, she saw her primary care physician who advised her to switch from her atenolol to alpha-methyl dopa (Aldomet), which she currently takes 250 mg TID. Her blood pressure now is 154/95. She has a mild headache, but no visual changes or abdominal discomfort. She does note some slight lower extremity edema. Which of the following is NOT a part of the management?

A. Change her Aldomet to labetalol.

B. Order LFTs, creatinine, and CBC.

C. She likely has preeclampsia and should be admitted to L&D.

D. Assess baseline creatinine clearance with a 24-hr urine protein.

E. Assess baseline proteinuria with a 24-hr collection.

QUESTION 44

A 24-year-old G2P0 woman presents at 17 weeks GA c/o increased vaginal discharge. She began noticing an increase in a clear, nonodorous discharge 2 days ago. She notes no fevers, chills, changes in bowel or urinary function, and no abdominal pain. She has had an uncomplicated pregnancy up to this point and had an elective termination of the last pregnancy at 12 weeks GA. On speculum exam, you note that the external os of the cervix looks slightly open, in addition to taking cultures and slide preparations of the vaginal discharge. There is no evidence for ruptured membranes, trichomoniasis, or bacterial vaginosis. You return to the bedside and perform a sterile vaginal exam. Her cervix is 1 cm dilated and 2 cm long. At this point, her management could include which of the following?

A. Oral metronidazole (Flagyl)

B. Cerclage placement

C. Amniocentesis for chromosomal abnormalities

D. Tocolysis with magnesium sulfate

E. Betamethasone for fetal lung maturity

QUESTION 45

A 23-year-old woman presents to your office with complaints of vulvar and vaginal pruritis. She became sexually active 2 weeks ago with a new partner and is concerned that this may be symptomatic of a sexually transmitted disease. She complains of an increase in a white, clumpy discharge without odor. She notes no abdominal pain or fever. On physical exam you note some erythematous punctate macular lesions bilaterally near the perineum, but no papular or vesicular lesions. On speculum exam, there is a white discharge that has a negative whiff test and on a KOH prepared slide reveals the image below: See Figure 45. What is the treatment of choice?

A. Oral acyclovir

B. Topical acyclovir applied to the lesions

C. Oral metronidazole (Flagyl)

D. Vaginal metronidazole (Metro-gel)

E. Oral fluconazole (Diflucan)

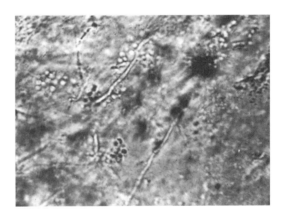

FIGURE 45

QUESTION 46

A 27-year-old attorney presents to your gynecology clinic for an annual exam. She has not had an exam for 3 years, but has never had any problems prior. She presents because she is interested in birth control as she is now in a monogamous sexual relationship. As part of this routine exam you perform a Pap smear, do testing for gonorrhea and chlamydia, and start her on a monophasic oral contraceptive pill. The Pap smear returns with a result of mild dysplasia/low-grade squamous intraepithelial lesion/CIN I. You meet with her 2 weeks later to discuss the ramifications of this finding. You tell her the following in your discussion:

A. With CIN I, the average length of time to the development of cervical cancer is 3–4 years.

B. Seventy percent of CIN I lesions resolve spontaneously.

C. The next step in management is cryotherapy.

D. Cervical dysplasia is highly associated with HPV subtypes 16 and 18.

E. The next step in management is laser therapy.

QUESTION 47

A couple presents to your office for an infertility evaluation. He is 48 and she is 33. He has conceived once 20 years ago, and she has never conceived. They have been trying to conceive for 15 months and have used the basal body temperature to show that she is ovulating in order to time intercourse the last 3 months. Among your early workup for this couple, you order a semen analysis on him and a day 21 progesterone on her. Which of the following is NOT routinely evaluated on semen analysis?

A. Semen ejaculate volume

B. Sperm motility

C. Semen pH

D. Sperm concentration in the semen

E. Semen chloride concentration

QUESTION 48

A couple presents to your infertility clinic. He is 33 and she is 27. They have been trying to conceive for 9 months, but report unprotected intercourse for more than 18 months. Both have conceived before. She had a pregnancy that resulted in a first-trimester miscarriage when she was 20, and he had a child and a termination of pregnancy with another partner 9 and 7 years ago, respectively. A semen analysis returns normal and a day 21 progesterone verifies that she is ovulating. The next testing ordered is a hysterosalpingogram to assess tubal patency. Which of the following would NOT be associated with tubal blockade or tubal dysfunction leading to infertility?

A. Prior pelvic inflammatory disease

B. Prior ectopic pregnancy

C. Prior use of the intrauterine device (IUD)

D. Endometriosis

E. Ruptured appendicitis

QUESTION 49

A 59-year-old G10P8 woman presents with complaints of new onset vaginal bleeding. She notes that bleeding started about a week ago with fresh bleeding and has reduced to brown spotting over the past few days. She denies cramping, abdominal pain or distension, and changes in weight. Her medical history is significant for type II diabetes for 7 years, hypertension, and obesity. She has a history of eight term vaginal deliveries and two spontaneous abortions. She underwent menopause at age 54 and has been on continuous combination estrogen/progesterone replacement over the past 5 years with no vaginal bleeding whatsoever over the past 4 years. You perform an endometrial biopsy, which returns as Grade I adenocarcinoma. Which of the following attributes of her history is NOT associated with endometrial cancer?

A. Diabetes

B. Hypertension

C. Late menopause

D. Obesity

E. Grand multiparity

QUESTION 50

A 63-year-old woman presents with complaints of leaking urine. She started noticing occasional leakage about 6 months ago, occurring approximately once or twice a week during physical activity (hiking or in her yoga class). Over the past month, however, she notes an increase in frequency, leaking small amounts of urine several times a day. She got an upper respiratory infection 2 weeks ago and noticed that she leaked urine whenever she coughed. She doesn't notice any leakage while she sleeps nor while she is seated, but will have a small leak when she rises from sitting. She denies dysuria or inability to control micturition if she feels a urinary urge.

Other past medical history reveals that she is a G5P4 with four vaginal deliveries. She went through menopause at age 51 and is not currently on HRT. On physical exam, you note mild uterine descensus and a grade I cystocele. A Q-tip test is positive, with an angle change from 10° to approximately 60°. See Figure 50. You tell her she most likely has

A. Stress incontinence

B. Urge incontinence

C. Detrusor instability

D. Total incontinence

E. Overflow incontinence

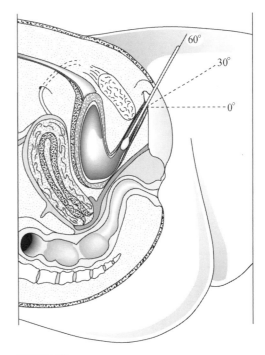

FIGURE 50

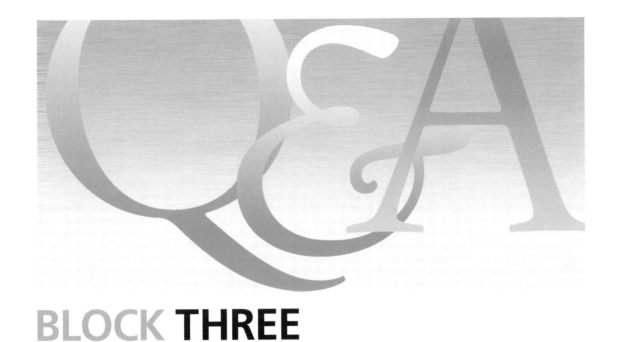

BLOCK THREE

QUESTIONS

Setting III: In-Patient Facilities

You have general admitting privileges to the hospital. You may see patients in the critical care unit or the pediatrics unit or the maternity unit or in recovery. You may also be called to see patients in the psychiatric unit. There is a short-stay unit for patients undergoing same-day operations or being held for observation. There are adjacent nursing home/extended-care facilities and a detoxification unit where you may see patients.

QUESTION 51

A 29-year-old G2P1 at $39^2/_7$ weeks GA presents in active labor. She has been contracting for 4 hr and on admission is contracting painfully every 2–3 min. Her cervix is 4 cm dilated and the fetal head is at −1 station. The fetal heart rate tracing is reassuring with a baseline in the 140s, moderate variability, and frequent accelerations up to the 160s lasting 15–30 sec. By Leopolds, the estimated fetal weight is 3500 g and the position is left occiput posterior (LOP). The patient's prior labor lasted 13 hr and culminated in a spontaneous vaginal delivery of a 7 lb 8 oz boy (3400 g) after a 60-min second stage. The patient progresses slowly in labor, dilating approximately 1 cm every 1–2 hr during the next 6 hr. When she is 8 cm dilated, she requests an epidural, which is placed without complication. Over the next 4 hr; the patient slowly changes to full dilation. On exam, she is fully dilated, +1 station, and LOT position. She begins the second stage. After pushing for 2 hr, she is +3 station and LOA position. She requests assistance with a forceps or vacuum delivery because of exhaustion. Which of the following is UNNECESSARY for a low forceps delivery of this fetus? See Figures 51A and 51B

A. Anesthesia

B. Knowledge of station at or beyond +2

C. An estimate of fetal weight that is not macrosomic

D. Direct occiput anterior presentation

E. Skilled operator

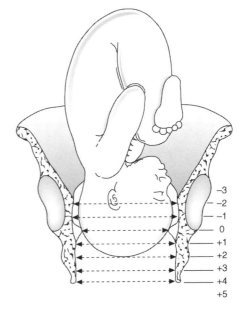

FIGURE 51A

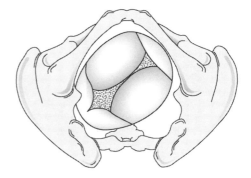

FIGURE 51B

QUESTION 52

A 46-year-old G0 obese woman with chronic hypertension and diabetes presents with infiltrating ductal carcinoma of the breast. She undergoes a wide local excision and axillary lymph-node dissection. Surgery is performed without complications and there is no evidence of metastatic disease on frozen section. You go to the postoperative area to discuss these findings with her. She is quite bitter about her diagnosis, but glad that she got the disease at age 46 rather than at age 42 like her sister who had bilateral disease requiring mastectomies. She asks you why she got breast cancer. You tell her which of the following was her strongest risk factor:

A.   Obesity

B.   Nulliparity

C.   Hypertension

D.   Family history

E.   Diabetes

QUESTION 53

A 53-year-old obese woman is undergoing a TAH-BSO for Stage I, Grade I endometrial cancer. During the case, a clamp on the left uterine artery slips and she loses a total of 1500 cc of blood during the case. Her preoperative hematocrit was 42. During the case, she received 3500 cc of crystalloid. At the end of the case, there was no obvious bleeding from this pedicle. Six hours postoperatively, she has a hematocrit drawn which returns 28. At this time, her blood pressure is 108/64 and her heart rate is 88. Her urine output over the prior 3 hr has been 55, 50, and 65 cc. What is the next step in management?

A.   Follow serial hematocrits

B.   This is an appropriate drop—check hematocrit in AM

C.   Immediate exploration

D.   Transfuse 2 units of PRBCs

E.   Check PT/PTT

QUESTION 54

A 19-year-old G1P0 at $39^5/_7$ GA presents with uterine contractions every 3–4 min. On exam, she is 4 cm dilated, 100% effaced, +1 station. She is admitted to labor and delivery, and over the next 2 hr her cervix changes to 6 cm dilation, +1 station, and left occiput anterior position (LOA). At this point, she requests an epidural. One hour after its placement, her exam is unchanged at 6 cm and +1 station. Artificial rupture of the membranes is performed and Pitocin is begun for augmentation of labor. Over the ensuing 2 hr, she contracts every 3–5 min and she changes to 7 cm and +1 station. After 2 more hr, she maintains the same exam of 7 cm and +1 station, with a position of LOA. At this point, the diagnosis of failure to progress in labor is suggested. Which of the following is most important to making this diagnosis?

A. Placement of an intrauterine pressure catheter to measure contractions

B. Cervical change of less than 1.5 cm per hour

C. At least 2 hr of Pitocin augmentation

D. No change in station over a period of 4 hr

E. An active phase of the second stage of labor greater than 5 hr

QUESTION 55

A 36-year-old G0 woman presents for operative hysteroscopy and resection of an intrauterine fibroid, which is the presumed cause of her infertility. During the case, the uterus is sounded to 7 cm. During dilation, you notice that dilation is quite difficult until, suddenly, the 7 French dilator passes easily, but to a distance of 10 cm. Presumably, you have perforated the uterus. The next step in management is:

A. Continue with the case

B. Proceed to exploratory laparotomy

C. Proceed to laparoscopy

D. Follow vital signs and order a pelvic ultrasound

E. As most of these perforations are not associated with morbidity, allow the patient to go home.

QUESTION 56

A 33-year-old G4P3 at term presents in active labor at 5-cm dilation. She has a reactive fetal heart tracing with a baseline in the 150s. Contractions are every 2–3 min. Estimated fetal weight is 3600 g and she had rupture of membranes approximately 3 hr prior to presentation. During the next hour, the fetal heart rate tracing begins to show decelerations. These decelerations begin about 30 sec after the contraction begins and end at about 30 sec after the contraction ends. See Figure 56. These decelerations are called _____ and are likely secondary to_____?

A. Early decelerations due to head compression

B. Variable decelerations due to uteroplacental insufficiency

C. Late decelerations due to uteroplacental insufficiency

D. Late decelerations due to head compression

E. Early decelerations due to a nuchal cord

QUESTION 57

A 19-year-old G1P0 at 41²/₇ weeks GA has just undergone a spontaneous vaginal delivery of a viable 4425-g boy. She had been diagnosed with preeclampsia and has been on magnesium sulfate for seizure prophylaxis for 26 hr. She spiked a fever to 101.8°F (38.8°C) 5 hr ago and is being treated with cefotetan for presumed chorioamnionitis. After the delivery of the placenta, which appears intact and without obvious vessels traveling into the membranes, she begins to have a postpartum hemorrhage. During the next minute she loses 300 cc of blood, for a total of approximately 800 cc. Which of the following is the most likely etiology in this clinical situation?

A. Cervical laceration

B. Vaginal laceration

C. Ruptured hemorrhoidal vessels

D. Uterine atony

E. Retained products of conception

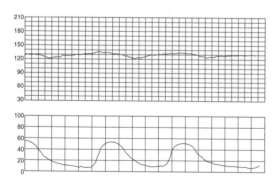

FIGURE 56

QUESTION 58

A 54-year-old woman presents for an exploratory laparotomy and TAH-BSO for a 7 cm left pelvic mass. Upon entering the abdomen, peritoneal washings are taken. The mass is isolated to the left ovary with no evidence that it is broken beyond the capsule. Upon examination of the uterus, tubes, and contralateral ovary, there is no gross evidence of disease. Upon palpation of the pelvic and aortic lymph nodes, they seem entirely normal. There is no evidence of any lesions on the bowel, omentum, or diaphragm either. Final pathology returns consistent with the above gross findings, but with positive malignant cells in the washings. Given the above tumor and the positive peritoneal washings, what is the stage of this ovarian cancer?

A. Ia

B. Ib

C. Ic

D. IIb

E. IIIc

QUESTION 59

A 17-year-old G1P0 at $37^2/_7$ weeks GA presents with blood pressures elevated to 146–158/93–102. A urine dipstick shows 2+ proteinuria. She denies headache or visual changes, but she does note some swelling of her hands. On physical exam, you note no papilledema, no right upper quadrant tenderness, brisk 3+ DTRs, and 2+ pitting edema of the lower extremities. She is admitted to labor and delivery, begun on magnesium sulfate for seizure prophylaxis, and her labor is induced. Which of the following lab tests is unnecessary?

A. Creatinine

B. CBC

C. AST

D. Uric acid

E. LDH or peripheral smear

QUESTION 60

A 32-year-old G2P1 presents at $36^4/_7$ weeks GA with a dichorionic/diamniotic twin gestation. Her twin gestation was diagnosed by ultrasound at 8 weeks GA. An anatomic survey and amniocentesis were performed at 17 weeks GA, both of which were normal. The fetal karyotypes are 46XY and 46XX. The patient had another ultrasound at 29 weeks GA, which showed concordant fetal growth with percentile weights of 46 and 57%, respectively. The patient now presents with contractions every 2–3 min and a cervical exam of 2 cm dilation, 90% effacement, and 0 station. You counsel her that which of the following is commonly accepted in the delivery of twins?

A. Trial of labor for breech presenting twin, cephalic second twin

B. High dose Pitocin after delivery of the first twin to remove the placenta

C. Immediate delivery of the second twin with forceps, despite the cervix being no longer fully dilated

D. Elective cesarean delivery for a cephalic presenting first twin and cephalic presenting second twin

E. After delivery of the first twin, immediate breech extraction of the second twin

QUESTION 61

A 32-year-old G0 patient is undergoing laparoscopy for evaluation of her infertility. A hysterosalpingogram (HSG) showed spillage from the left side, but only partial filling on the right. The patient has no history of pelvic pain or dysmenorrhea. In addition, she has regular menses and a positive LH spike on Day 13 of her cycle. On entering the abdomen, you notice extensive pelvic adhesions and a 3–4 cm endometrioma on the right ovary. The right adnexa is adherent to the right pelvic sidewall. When the uterus is injected with indigo-carmen dye, there is spillage from both sides, left first and then a small trickle from the right. The patient's etiology of her infertility is

A. Chronic PID leading to lack of tubal patency

B. Endometriosis leading to lack of tubal patency

C. Endometriosis leading to ovarian dysfunction

D. Endometriosis with uncertain pathophysiology

E. Uncertain etiology leading to lack of tubal patency

QUESTION 62

A 47-year-old woman undergoes a radical hysterectomy and bilateral salpingo-oophorectomy for Stage Ib cervical carcinoma. At the beginning of the case, compression stockings and pneumoboots are placed for DVT prophylaxis. During the case, she has an estimated blood loss of 750 cc. At the end of the case, you are writing orders. In addition to pneumoboots, which of the following is most commonly used for DVT prophylaxis in postoperative patients with cancer?

A. Coumadin

B. Heparin SQ 5000 units TID

C. LMW heparin SQ 40 units QD

D. LMW heparin SQ 40 units BID

E. Anticoagulation is not given postoperatively

QUESTION 63

A 28-year-old G3P2 at $38^2/_7$ weeks GA presents in active labor, 4 cm dilated, 90% effaced, and +1 station. The fetus is breech. The fetus had been breech 2 weeks earlier. An attempt at external version failed. CT for pelvimetry found the pelvis to be adequate for breech delivery. After a discussion of the risks and benefits of breech delivery with her primary obstetrician, the patient elected to attempt a trial of labor. See Figure 63. Which of the following is NOT generally considered necessary in the decision to allow a trial of labor for a breech presenting fetus?

A. Estimated fetal weight less than 4000 g

B. Breech is either complete or frank

C. Fetal head is flexed

D. Lack of known fetal anomalies

E. Patient has an epidural for anesthesia

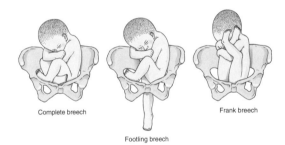

Complete breech

Footling breech

Frank breech

FIGURE 63

QUESTION 64

A 22-year-old G1P0 at 29^2/$_7$ weeks GA presents with complaints of recurrent lower back pain. She is placed on the fetal heart monitor and tocometer and is found to be contracting every 2–3 min. She has no complaints of fluid leakage, though notes she had some spotting the last time she urinated. A sterile speculum is negative for pooling, nitrazine, and ferning. On exam, she is 2 cm dilated, 85% effaced, at +1 station and cephalic presenting. Which of the following would NOT be part of her management?

A. A 6 g IV bolus of magnesium sulfate

B. A bolus of IV penicillin

C. A 12 mg IM dose of betamethasone

D. A 500 mg IV bolus of erythromycin

E. Culture of the perineum and vagina for group B streptococcus (GBS)

QUESTION 65

A 37-year-old woman is undergoing a TAH–BSO for chronic pelvic pain from Stage IV endometriosis. There is extensive dissection to free the left adnexa from the bowel and from the pelvic sidewalls. Identification of the ureter on the left side is adequate. However, the right ureter is difficult to identify above the pelvic brim. At one point in the case there is a question of right ureteral injury. After the specimen is removed, indigo-carmine dye is given IV and spills out of the right ureter approximately 4 cm above the pelvic brim. The distal portion is easily identified and there is no obviously missing portion. The best repair of this injury is:

A. End-to-end reanastomosis

B. End-to-side reanastomosis

C. Ureteral reimplantation into the bladder dome

D. Ureteral reimplantation into the contralateral ureter

E. Cannot be repaired—place nephrostomy tube

QUESTION 66

A 62-year-old woman is admitted for exploratory laparotomy and debulking procedure for likely ovarian cancer. Upon entering the abdomen, there is bulky disease on every peritoneal surface and surrounding much of the bowel and omentum (a "peek and shriek" case). No further surgical intervention is undertaken and the patient is closed, and subsequently admitted postoperatively to the gyn-oncology service for her first round of chemotherapy. Her chemotherapeutic regimen should consist of:

A. CHOP (cyclophosphamide, doxorubicin, Oncovin, prednisone)

B. Taxol and carboplatin

C. Melphalan

D. Etoposide and cisplatin

E. CMF (cyclophosphamide, methotrexate, fluorouracil)

QUESTION 67

A 31-year-old G2P1 patient at $39^{2}/_{7}$ weeks GA presents complaining of leaking clear fluid for the last hour. One hour prior to presenting, she had a large gush of about 100 cc of fluid, and has had smaller leaks since then. She has had no contractions or bleeding. On sterile speculum exam, you note a small pool of clear fluid in the vagina. A sample of this fluid is nitrazine positive and ferns when dried on a slide. On inspection, the cervix is long and closed. The fetal heart rate tracing is reactive and without decelerations. Which of the following is NOT a reasonable approach to management based on existing literature?

A. Immediate induction of labor with oxytocin

B. Expectant management for the next 12 hr, then induction if no signs of labor

C. Immediate induction of labor with prostaglandins

D. Expectant management at home for the next 24 hr

E. Expectant management at home for the next 96 hr

QUESTION 68

A 26-year-old G1P0 presents in active labor at 39²/₇ weeks GA. She had an uncomplicated antepartum course and has a history of scleroderma. Her disease is currently under control with the use of prednisone. In labor, you begin stress dose steroids. Two hours later, you are called by nursing for a prolonged deceleration. Upon pelvic examination, you note a prolapsed umbilical cord beyond the fetal head. You lift the fetal head off of the cord and the fetal heart rate returns to the 130s. The patient is moved to the operating room for an emergent cesarean delivery as you continue to lift the fetal head off the umbilical cord. In the OR, the obstetric anesthesiologist asks about your preference for anesthesia. You say that:

A. Epidural anesthesia is preferred.

B. Spinal anesthesia is preferred.

C. She needs to be given general anesthesia.

D. You can use local anesthesia with conscious sedation.

E. A pudendal block can be placed.

QUESTION 69

A 23-year-old patient presents 2 days post-op with complaints of abdominal pain and fever. She had undergone a laparoscopic resection and fulguration of endometriosis with unipolar cautery. She is seen in the ED by her primary physician. On physical examination, she has a temperature of 101.4°F (38.6°C), tachycardia to 120s, and an abdominal exam with rebound tenderness. Her bimanual exam has some slight cervical motion tenderness. She is given the diagnosis of postoperative pelvic inflammatory disease. She is admitted to the Gyn floor and started on triple antibiotics. Three hours after admission, you are consulted because her abdominal pain is increasing, her blood pressure is now 80/40, and her heart rate is in the 130s. Her abdomen is diffusely tender with rebound in all quadrants. The most likely etiology of her symptoms and signs is:

A. Postoperative PID

B. Endomyometritis

C. Appendicitis

D. Ureteral injury

E. Bowel injury

QUESTION 70

A 23-year-old G1P0 presents in active labor. She progresses rapidly to complete dilation and undergoes a 30-min second stage. She delivers a viable fetus with apgars of 8 and 9. Upon inspection of the fetus, you note that the infant has either an enlarged clitoris or a very small penis, and partially fused labioscrotal swellings. You order a 17-hydroxyprogesterone, which is elevated. In addition to telling the patient and her husband the likely sex of the child, you also mention that which of the following treatments will be necessary in this patient?

A. Immediate surgery to correct the genitalia

B. Estradiol

C. Progesterone

D. Testosterone

E. Prednisone

QUESTION 71

A 31-year-old G2P1 presents in active labor at $39^5/_7$ weeks GA. She is 5 cm dilated, 90% effaced, and +1 station. The fetal heart rate tracing is reassuring with no decelerations, and the tocometer reveals contractions every 2–3 min. She has had an uncomplicated prenatal course. Her obstetrical history is remarkable for a cesarean delivery 4 years ago with failure to progress past 7 cm dilation. On labor and delivery, she requests an epidural, which is placed without complication. On her next examination, 2 hr later, she is 7 cm dilated and +2 station, but her contractions have decreased to every 5–7 min. She is begun on oxytocin for augmentation. An hour-and-a-half later, the nurse calls you for a prolonged fetal heart rate deceleration. She has already stopped the Pitocin, given oxygen by facemask, and changed the patient's position. The heart rate had dropped from a baseline in the 150s to the 70s and now, after 4 min, is coming back above the 120s. Looking at the monitor strip for the prior 30 min, you note repetitive variable decelerations that last 30–40 sec and contractions every 2–3 min. On examination, the cervix is 8–9 cm dilated, but the fetal head cannot be easily palpated, indicating that it is at least above −3 station. The next step in management of this patient is:

A. Apply fetal scalp electrode

B. Cesarean delivery

C. Forceps delivery

D. Expectant management

E. Restart Pitocin to help bring the head back down.

QUESTION 72

A 17-year-old G0 patient presents to the ED with complaints of fever and lower abdominal pain. On physical exam she has a temperature of 101.2°F (38.4°C) and bilateral lower abdominal tenderness. On bimanual exam she has cervical motion tenderness with bilateral adnexal tenderness. There is a slight fullness on her right that is difficult to assess because of her discomfort. She is admitted to the hospital with the diagnosis of PID and started on cefoxitin and doxycycline. After 48 hr of this therapy, she still has fevers to 101.6°F (38.7°C). The next step in management is:

A. Laparoscopy

B. Laparotomy

C. Await final cultures

D. Pelvic ultrasound

E. Change antibiotics to ampicillin and gentamicin

QUESTION 73

A 33-year-old G4P2 patient at $38^{5}/_{7}$ weeks GA has been in the second stage of labor for 3 hr when you are called for the delivery. She presented with contractions about 12 hr ago and was 3 cm dilated. She made reasonable progress, becoming fully dilated over the ensuing 10 hr with oxytocin augmentation. Her antenatal course was complicated only by diet-controlled gestational diabetes. Her last two births were 7 and 5 years ago, both vaginal, with fetal weights of 8.5 and 9 lb, respectively. As the fetus is beginning to crown, you are prepared to:

A. Perform a forceps delivery

B. Perform a vacuum delivery

C. Perform a cesarean delivery

D. Manage a shoulder dystocia

E. Manage a uterine inversion

QUESTION 74

A 57-year-old woman underwent a total abdominal hysterectomy and bilateral salpingo-oophorectomy with bilateral pelvic lymph node sampling for Stage I, Grade III endometrial cancer. She was discharged home on postoperative day three with oral cephalexin (Keflex) because of a wound cellulitis. She now returns 2 days later with complaints of leaking pus from the lateral edge of the incision. On physical exam she is obese, with a Pfannenstiel skin incision that has surrounding erythema 3–4 cm superiorly. The left aspect of the incision is slightly open, and when you palpate the area a small amount of thick yellowish discharge is extruded. You attempt to probe the incision with a cotton swab, but it cannot be passed into the small opening. Your next step is:

A. Start the patient on intravenous antibiotics.

B. Schedule the patient for an incision and drainage of the wound in the OR.

C. Using local anesthesia, open the lateral edge of the incision with a scalpel for further exploration.

D. Using an IV catheter, irrigate the small opening at the lateral edge of the incision.

E. Order a CT scan to examine the incision.

QUESTION 75

A 66-year-old woman is 12 hr post-op from an exploratory laparotomy and debulking procedure for ovarian cancer. At the time of the surgery, approximately 4 l of ascites were removed from the abdomen. You are called by nursing because the patient has made only 15 cc of urine over the last hour. While examining her fluid intake and output for the day, you note that she received 1600 cc of fluid intraoperatively and 100 cc per hour since. In the OR her blood loss was 700 cc and urine output 200 cc for the 3-hr case. Postoperatively, she has put out a total of 520 cc of urine, but the past 3 hr have been 30, 25, and 15 cc, respectively. In addition, she has had 250 cc of serosanguinous fluid drained from two intraabdominal drains. The next step in management is:

Table:	In	Out
OR	1600 cc crystalloid	700 cc EBL, 200 cc urine
Post-op	1200 cc crystalloid	520 cc urine, 250 from drains Past 3 hr 30/25/15

A. Bolus 500 cc IV crystalloid

B. Bolus 2000 cc IV crystalloid

C. Bolus IV colloid, salt poor albumin

D. Give IV furosemide (Lasix)

E. Give PO furosemide (Lasix)

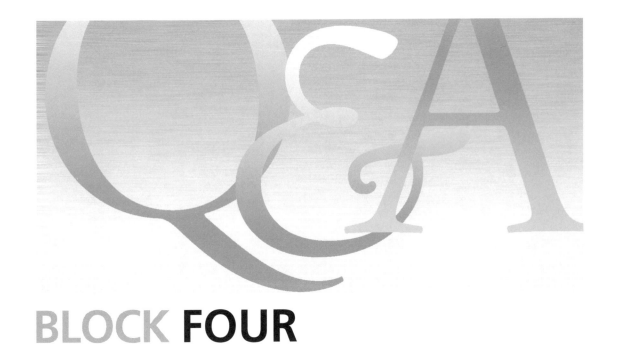

BLOCK **FOUR**

QUESTIONS

Setting IV: Emergency Department

Generally, patients encountered here are seeking urgent care and most are not known to you. Available to you are a full range of social services, including rape crisis intervention, family support, child protective services, domestic violence support, psychiatric services, and security assistance backed up by local police. Complete laboratory and radiology services are available.

QUESTION 76

A 33-year-old G3P2 woman who had an uncomplicated delivery of an infant 3 weeks ago presents to the ED complaining of right breast pain and fever for 2 days. On physical exam, you note an area of focal tenderness, warmth, and erythema on the right breast. The patient is found to have a temperature of 101.2°F (38.4°C) and an elevated white blood cell count of 12,000. All of the following are appropriate treatment recommendations for mastitis EXCEPT:

A. Symptomatic treatment of pain with NSAIDs

B. Dicloxacillin for 7–10 days

C. Keflex for 7–10 days

D. Warm compresses on the affected breast

E. Stop breast-feeding until completion of antibiotic course

QUESTION 77

A 23-year-old G0 woman presents with acute onset, severe right lower quadrant pain, and mild nausea. She denies fever, chills, vaginal bleeding, or discharge, and reports feeling this pain twice in the last 6 months with this time being the worst it has ever been. On physical exam, she is afebrile, appears extremely uncomfortable, and has severe RLQ tenderness, but does not have any peritoneal signs. Pelvic exam is significant for a tender right adnexal mass and cervical motion tenderness. Pelvic ultrasound reveals minimal fluid in the cul-de-sac and a 6-cm

right adnexal mass with no Doppler flow. See Figure 77. Her white blood cell count and hematocrit are normal, and a urine pregnancy test is negative. Which of the following is the most likely diagnosis?

A. Acute appendicitis

B. Early ectopic pregnancy

C. Torsion of adnexa

D. Pelvic inflammatory disease

E. Ruptured hemorrhagic ovarian cyst

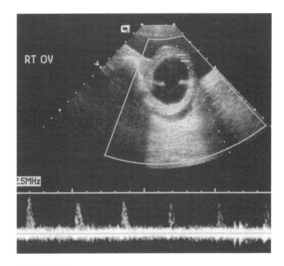

FIGURE 77

QUESTION 78

A 27-year-old G1P0 woman presents to the ED with complaints of heavy vaginal bleeding and painful abdominal cramping that started this morning. She reports that she stopped taking birth control pills approximately 3 months ago in an effort to conceive, and had some light spotting a month later, but no normal menstrual period since that time. Her blood type is O positive and her hematocrit is 39.2. A urine pregnancy test in the ED is positive. On physical exam, you note mild lower abdominal tenderness in the midline, but an otherwise benign abdominal exam. On speculum exam, you note a large amount of bright red blood in the vaginal vault and an open cervical os containing large blood clots. Endovaginal ultrasound confirms the presence of a gestational sac in the uterus consistent with a 6-week gestation, but no yolk sac is visible. See Figure 78. What is the correct diagnosis and management of this patient?

A. Ectopic pregnancy, managed by emergent surgery

B. Threatened abortion, managed by dilatation and curettage

C. Incomplete abortion, expectant management

D. Inevitable abortion, managed by dilatation and curettage

E. Complete abortion, expectant management

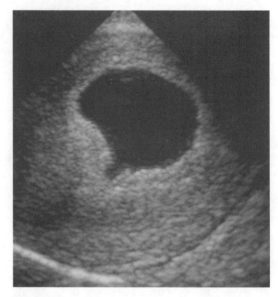

FIGURE 78

QUESTION 79

A 62-year-old G0 woman presents to the ED complaining of 2 weeks of vaginal spotting. She denies trauma or recent intercourse. Of note, she experienced menopause at age 52, has never been on hormone replacement, and her last Pap smear 3 months ago was normal. On physical exam, she is found to be obese, and pelvic exam reveals an atrophic vagina, a normal-appearing cervix, and a minimal amount of blood in the vaginal vault with no evidence of active bleeding. Her hematocrit is 29 and an endovaginal ultrasound reveals an 8-mm thick endometrial lining. Which of the following is the next appropriate step in evaluating vaginal bleeding in a postmenopausal woman?

A. Pap smear to rule out cervical etiologies

B. Endometrial biopsy to assess the endometrium

C. Hysteroscopy to search for potential causes of bleeding

D. Dilation and curettage

E. Prescribe hormone replacement to stop the bleeding

QUESTION 80

A 19-year-old G0 woman presents to the ED several hours after experiencing a sudden sharp pain in the left lower quadrant that has subsided over the last few hours and become more diffuse. Her last menstrual period was approximately 2 weeks ago. She reports similar prior episodes of pain on the right side 2–3 months ago, has been sexually active with the same partner for 2 years, and denies vaginal discharge. She is afebrile, has a normal white count, and a negative urine pregnancy test. On physical exam, she has mild diffuse abdominal pain, but no peritoneal signs. Pelvic exam is within normal limits with no cervical motion tenderness. What is the most likely diagnosis?

A. Mittelschmerz

B. Pelvic inflammatory disease

C. Adnexal torsion

D. Ruptured ectopic pregnancy

E. Appendicitis

QUESTION 81

A 20-year-old G2P1 woman presents to the ED complaining of nausea, vomiting, and lower abdominal pain for the past 2 days. She reports intermittent condom usage with her partner of 3 months. Her vital signs are within normal limits, with the exception of a temperature of 100.2°F (37.9°C). On exam, you note abdominal, adnexal, and cervical motion tenderness, but no peritoneal signs. There is mucopurulent discharge noted at the cervical os. A urine pregnancy test is negative, and her white blood cell count is 9700/mm^3. A wet mount shows numerous leukocytes. All of the following are criteria for inpatient treatment of PID EXCEPT:

A. Pregnancy

B. Severe nausea and vomiting

C. Age less than 40

D. Failure of outpatient therapy

E. Unreliable patient

QUESTION 82

A 22-year-old G1P0 woman presents to the ED approximately 40 hr after experiencing a condom failure. She is anxious and requesting emergency contraception. You prescribe two 50 μg birth control pills now and another two to be taken in 12 hr. Which of the following statements regarding emergency contraception is FALSE:

A. Emergency contraception is not effective if greater than 48 hr have passed since the time of unprotected intercourse.

B. A pregnancy test should be performed prior to prescribing emergency contraception.

C. Nausea is a common side effect due to the high doses of hormones in emergency contraception.

D. Patients should be advised to seek medical attention including pregnancy testing if menses has not begun within 21 days of treatment.

E. Emergency contraception can also be obtained by danazol, antiprogestins, synthetic and conjugated estrogens, and the insertion of an intrauterine device (IUD).

QUESTION 83

A 28-year-old G3P0 woman is brought to the ED shortly after passing out. She is conscious on arrival, but appears to be in acute distress and severe pain. She reports vaginal bleeding and worsening left lower abdominal pain that became sharp and severe just prior to her loss of consciousness. She had a positive urine pregnancy test 4 weeks ago and is certain that her last menstrual period was 10 weeks ago. Past medical history is significant for pelvic inflammatory disease that was treated 5 years ago. Her vital signs are BP 92/60, pulse 118, respirations 26, and temperature 97.2°F (36.2°C). Urine pregnancy test is positive. The patient has a normal white blood cell count and a hematocrit of 32.3. On physical exam, she has diffuse lower abdominal pain and exhibits guarding. Pelvic exam reveals cervical motion tenderness and significant tenderness to palpation in the left adnexal region. Transvaginal ultrasound shows a large amount of free fluid in the cul-de-sac, but no masses and no intrauterine pregnancy. See Figure 83. What is the most appropriate next step in managing this patient?

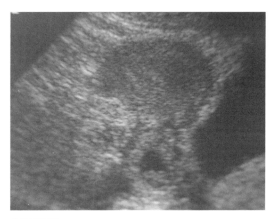

FIGURE 83

A. Uterine curettage to definitively exclude ectopic pregnancy.

B. Perform a culdocentesis.

C. Obtain a quantitative beta-hCG level to determine whether medical or surgical treatment is indicated.

D. Administer methotrexate and follow serial quantitative beta-hCG levels for appropriate decline.

E. Stabilize the patient and take her emergently to the operating room.

QUESTION 84

A 20-year-old G0 woman presents to the ED in tears. She reports being sexually assaulted by three men unknown to her while attending a party this evening. You obtain a history from her, which is difficult because she is visibly shaken and upset. She doesn't believe any of the assailants used a condom and is unsure whether they ejaculated. There was no oral or anal penetration. On speculum examination, you obtain swabs from the vagina for evidence and for microscopic examination. You do not see any evidence of spermatozoa, Trichomonads, or bacterial vaginosis. Which of the following would be INCORRECT management of this patient?

A. Ovral (ethinyl estradiol 50 mcg, and norgestrel 0.5 mg) 2 tablets Q 12 hr PO × 2 doses

B. Azithromycin 1 g PO and Ceftriaxone 250 mg IM × 1

C. Contact police despite her objections.

D. Reassure her that she has no risk of pregnancy.

E. Offer baseline HIV testing and AZT prophylaxis.

QUESTION 85

A 17-year-old G0 woman is brought to the ED by her mother who is concerned that the patient has been experiencing fevers, rigors, nausea, vomiting, and myalgias since this morning. She is not sexually active, and her last menstrual period began 5 days ago. Her vital signs are BP 84/51, T 103.1°F (39.5°C), P 122, and R 24. On physical exam, the patient appears acutely ill, has a diffuse erythematous rash, and mild, diffuse abdominal tenderness, but no nuchal rigidity. After removal of a blood-saturated tampon, pelvic exam reveals a small amount of blood in the vaginal vault but no cervical motion tenderness or vaginal discharge, and the uterus and adnexa are within normal limits. Laboratory studies are significant for a white blood cell count of 16,000, platelets of 93,000, and elevated BUN and creatinine. Which of the following statements about this patient's diagnosis is FALSE?

A. It is caused by *Staphylococcus aureus*.

B. It has been associated with polycystic ovarian syndrome (PCOS), vaginal infections, vaginal and cesarean delivery, and postpartum endometritis.

C. Blood cultures are often negative.

D. Treatment may include admission to an intensive care unit for management of hypotension.

E. There are approximately 200 cases per year in the United States.

QUESTION 86

A 27-year-old G2P1 woman at 35^1/$_7$ weeks GA presents to OB triage and anxiously states that she has not felt the baby move for the past 5 hr. She denies vaginal bleeding, rupture of membranes, and uterine contractions. The pregnancy is complicated by poorly controlled gestational diabetes mellitus requiring insulin administration. The patient began twice weekly antepartum testing at 32 weeks GA, but has missed several appointments. Physical exam is significant for an obese woman with a random blood glucose of 154. Her cervical exam is 1 cm dilated, 50% effaced, and −3 station. Non-stress testing reveals a nonreactive fetal heart rate tracing and no uterine contractions. What is the most appropriate next step in the management of this high-risk patient with decreased fetal movement?

A. Administration of insulin to decrease the patient's glucose level

B. Vibroacoustic stimulation (VAS) of the fetus followed by ultrasound to look for gross and fine fetal movements

C. Administer betamethasone to promote fetal lung maturity in anticipation of possible premature delivery.

D. Begin induction of labor with a prostaglandin agent.

E. Emergent cesarean section

QUESTION 87

A 32-year-old G3P3 woman presents to the ED complaining of persistent fevers and abdominal pain that have worsened over the past day and are only temporarily relieved by ibuprofen. She is postpartum day 7 after a vaginal delivery of a term gestation infant male weighing 3500 g. The delivery was complicated by a postpartum hemorrhage requiring manual extraction of the placenta. Her vaginal bleeding has decreased since discharge from the hospital, requiring two to four pad changes per day. Her vital signs are BP 108/72, T 102.6°F (39.2°C), P 96, and R 20. On physical exam, she has fundal tenderness but no peritoneal signs. Pelvic exam confirms uterine tenderness and reveals scant vaginal bleeding as well as a minimal amount of purulent discharge. The laceration repair is intact and hemostatic. Laboratory studies reveal a hematocrit of 34.4 and a white blood cell count of 18,000 with a left shift. What is the appropriate diagnosis and treatment for this patient?

A. Delayed postpartum hemorrhage, dilatation and curettage

B. Placenta accreta, exploratory laparotomy

C. Undiagnosed vaginal hematoma, ligation of the offending blood vessel

D. Endomyometritis, clindamycin and gentamicin

E. Endomyometritis, dilation and curettage

QUESTION 88

A 28-year-old G0 woman presents to the ED after an episode of postcoital bleeding that soaked a pad over the last 2 hr. She reports approximately 4–5 prior episodes of postcoital bleeding over the last few months that were less severe. She denies any past medical history. Her menses occur every month and are regular. She has not had a Pap smear since age 18 when she first became sexually active. At that time, she was found to have chlamydia for which she underwent treatment. She reports multiple current sexual partners, and she uses condoms intermittently. Her hematocrit is 40.1. Vital signs and physical exam are within normal limits. Pelvic exam reveals a minimal amount of blood and watery discharge in the vaginal vault, and a 2×3 cm exophytic mass on the cervix that does not appear to involve the upper vagina or fornix. The uterus and adnexa are within normal limits. You biopsy the lesion, which returns 1 week later as cervical cancer invasive to 7 mm. The patient undergoes staging, which reveals negative cystoscopy, proctoscopy, and IVP. What is the stage and appropriate treatment of her disease?

A. Ib1, cone biopsy to preserve fertility

B. Ib1, radical hysterectomy or radiation therapy

C. Ib2, radical hysterectomy or radiation therapy

D. IIa, radical hysterectomy

E. IIb, radiation therapy

QUESTION 89

A 34-year-old G4P3 woman at $33^4/_7$ weeks GA presents to the ED complaining of a gush of vaginal bleeding as well as the onset of severely painful uterine contractions. The patient denies history of abdominal trauma, recent intercourse, or cocaine usage. Her vital signs are BP 162/99, T 98.4°F (36.9°C), P 114, and R 18. Physical exam reveals a woman in moderate distress with a firm and tender uterus. The fetal heart rate (FHR) tracing is initially formally reactive with a baseline rate of approximately 140 beats per minutes (bpm). Ultrasound examination confirms that there is no evidence of placenta previa. On sterile speculum exam, there is a moderate amount of blood in the vaginal vault. Cervical exam reveals $1^1/_2$ cm dilation, 50% effacement, and −3 station. As you are writing her note, the nurse informs you that the FHR tracing now shows a prolonged deceleration of 5 min to approximately 80 bpm with no signs of spontaneous recovery to baseline. See Figure 89. The nurse has already turned the patient to her left side, given O_2 by facemask, and checked her BP, which is 158/102. What is the most appropriate next step in management?

A. Transfuse two units PRBCs immediately and have the lab type and cross two additional units.

B. Administer betamethasone to promote fetal lung maturity in anticipation of preterm delivery.

C. Administer magnesium sulfate tocolysis to alleviate the fetal distress from contractions.

D. Initiate induction of labor for nonreassuring FHR tracing.

E. Move to the OR for cesarean section for nonreassuring FHR tracing.

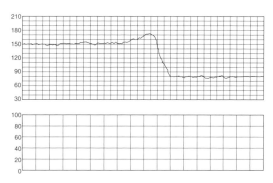

FIGURE 89

QUESTION 90

A 36-year-old G2P2 woman presents to the ED with acute onset shortness of breath and chest pain. She is 3 days postpartum following an uncomplicated delivery. Of note, the patient is not breast-feeding. She denies a history of trauma. Her past medical history is significant for obesity, and her vital signs are BP 116/74, T 100.0°F (37.7°C), P 112, RR 28, and O_2 sat 91% RA. On physical exam, she is in moderate distress, tachypneic, and has rales and mildly decreased breath sounds in the left lung. Pelvic exam reveals a minimal amount of blood in the vaginal vault but is otherwise within normal limits. Chest x-ray is negative, but EKG reveals sinus tachycardia and nonspecific ST-T changes. A blood gas drawn on room air reveals an a-A gradient of 43. You order a ventilation–perfusion (V-Q) scan, which is read as inconclusive. At this point, a pulmonary angiogram is performed. See Figure 90. Which of the following would be an inappropriate treatment for this patient?

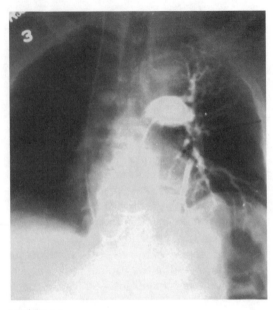

FIGURE 90

A. Supplemental oxygen to achieve arterial oxygen tension of ≥70 mm Hg

B. Heparin 10,000 unit bolus followed by 1000 units per hour until the partial thromboplastin time (PTT) is 2.5–3 times normal

C. Low molecular weight heparin

D. Conversion from heparin to warfarin therapy to achieve INR of 2.0–3.0

E. None of the above

QUESTION 91

A 68-year-old G0 woman with a history of Stage IIIc ovarian cancer is brought to the ED by her daughter who states that the patient has had persistent nausea and vomiting for several days. She has not had anything to eat or drink for 2 days. Additionally, she has not had a bowel movement or passed gas in 5 days. Approximately 7 months ago, she underwent TAH-BSO, complete staging workup, and six cycles of chemotherapy for her ovarian cancer. Her vital signs are BP 114/72, T 100.8°F (38.2°C), P 108, and R 18. On physical exam, she is a thin, obtunded woman with dry mucous membranes and skin tenting. Abdominal exam reveals distention, absent bowel sounds, severe tenderness, and peritoneal signs. Laboratory studies are significant for a hematocrit of 48.2 and WBC of 15,000. You send the patient for KUB and upright x-rays, which reveal numerous air-fluid level and a sliver of hyperlucency below the diaphragm. Which is the next step in the management of this patient?

A. Insert a nasogastric tube (NGT) and expectant management

B. Begin total parenteral nutrition (TPN)

C. Laparoscopy to look for residual disease

D. Administer broad-spectrum antibiotics and plan laparotomy when her signs of infection have resolved

E. Proceed to the operating room for exploratory laparotomy

QUESTION 92

A 36-year-old G0 presents to the ED complaining of severe pelvic pain for 2 days. The patient is well known to you and has endometriosis confirmed by laparoscopy. She denies history of current or past physical or sexual abuse and does not desire future fertility. Over the past 3 years, she has tried various treatment regimens, including both cyclic and continuous oral contraceptives (OCPs), the latter yielding a 4-month pain-free period. The patient admits to recent discontinuation of the continuous OCPs secondary to concern regarding amenorrhea. Her vital signs are stable, and she is afebrile. Physical exam reveals normal bowel sounds, mild pelvic tenderness, but no masses or peritoneal signs. On pelvic exam, the patient has diffuse pelvic tenderness and uterosacral nodularity on rectovaginal exam. There are no adnexal masses, vaginal discharge, or bleeding. Pelvic ultrasound is within normal limits. What is the appropriate treatment for this patient?

A. Resume cyclic OCPs

B. Resume continuous OCPs

C. Trial of progestin treatment

D. Trial of GnRH agonist treatment

E. Exploratory laparoscopy

QUESTION 93

An 18-year-old G1P0 at $14^{4}/_{7}$ weeks GA presents to the ED complaining of weight loss and severe nausea and vomiting for 3 days. This is her fifth visit to the ED for this problem, and she has had two prior short-term hospitalizations. She has tried vitamin B6, Reglan, Tigan, and Compazine with only temporary relief. She has no significant past medical history, but is currently in an abusive relationship with the father of the baby. Her vital signs are BP 102/68, T 96.8°F (36°C), P 96, and R 16. On physical exam, she appears uncomfortable, has dry mucous membranes, and poor skin turgor. Pelvic exam is within normal limits. Laboratory studies reveal hypokalemia, hypochloremia, alkalemia, hematocrit of 48, and her BUN/creatinine ratio is >20:1. Urinalysis reveals ketones and high specific gravity. Which of the following would be the LAST step in management of this patient?

A. Hospitalization for IV hydration and repletion of electrolytes

B. Social work consultation

C. Zofran 4 mg IV, then 8 mg PO TID when tolerating POs

D. Initiation of total parenteral nutrition

E. Placement of NG feeding tube

QUESTION 94

A 17-year-old G3P0-1-1-1 at $32^{5}/_{7}$ weeks GA presents to the ED complaining of moderately painful uterine contractions every 5 min for the past hour. Significant prenatal issues include obesity (prepregnancy weight of 213 lb), history of a prior preterm delivery at 32 weeks GA, and history of a therapeutic abortion at 11 weeks GA 3 years ago. Her vital signs are stable, and she is afebrile. On physical exam, she is an obese woman in moderate discomfort but with an otherwise negative exam. Sterile speculum exam and wet mount reveal abundant pseudohyphae, and cervical exam reveals 3 cm dilation and 75% effacement. Which of the following is this patient's biggest risk factor for preterm delivery?

A. Prior preterm delivery

B. Prior therapeutic abortion (TAB)

C. Vaginal candidiasis

D. Prepregnancy weight

E. Maternal age

QUESTION 95

A 31-year-old G2P2 woman presents to the ED complaining of severe abdominal pain and vaginal spotting. She denies fever, chills, nausea, and vomiting. Over the past 6 months, she has noticed that the duration and amount of her regular menses has diminished. This is coincident with the fact that approximately 6 months ago, she underwent a LEEP (loop electrosurgical excision procedure) for cervical dysplasia. Her vital signs and physical exam are within normal limits. However, on pelvic exam, you note a slightly tender, anteverted, and anteflexed uterus with cervical motion tenderness and no cervical, uterine, or adnexal masses. Which of the following is the most likely diagnosis and appropriate treatment?

A. Pelvic abscess; CT-guided drainage

B. Endometriosis; exploratory laparoscopy

C. Progression of residual cervical dysplasia to cancer; hysterectomy

D. Cervical stenosis; oral contraceptives

E. Cervical stenosis; cervical dilatation

QUESTION 96

A 31-year-old G0 woman presents to the ED complaining of gradual onset left lower quadrant pain. She denies nausea, vomiting, fever, chills, constipation, or loose stools. However, she notes an 8-lb weight gain over the past month. Her gynecological history is significant for current infertility treatment by ovulation induction with gonadotropins. On infertility workup, she had a hysterosalpingogram that revealed an occluded left tube, and laparoscopy revealed Stage 3 endometriosis. The patient reports that she has continued to have unprotected intercourse throughout her current treatment. Her vital signs are within normal limits. On physical exam, you note mild abdominal distention, tenderness to palpation in the left lower quadrant, and a left adnexal mass. There is no blood or discharge in the vaginal vault, and no cervical motion tenderness. Ultrasound examination reveals an enlarged ovary approximately 7×8 cm in size and composed of numerous enlarged follicles. There is no free fluid in the cul-de-sac. Her hematocrit is 42 and white blood cell count 8000. The patient's most likely diagnosis is

A. Adnexal torsion

B. Ovarian hyperstimulation

C. Early ectopic pregnancy

D. Endometrioma

E. Pelvic inflammatory disease

QUESTION 97

A 24-year-old G1P0 who had a positive urine pregnancy test 9 weeks ago presents to the ED complaining of severe nausea, vomiting, and painless vaginal bleeding. She has not had her initial prenatal exam yet. She denies any significant past medical history. On physical exam, she has no abdominal tenderness, but her fundus is palpable just below the umbilicus. Pelvic exam reveals a small amount of tissue at the cervical os, but no lesion, discharge, or active bleeding. Quantitative beta-hCG is 117,000. Ultrasound examination reveals a "snow storm" pattern, no fetal heart sounds, and no evidence of an intrauterine pregnancy. See Figure 97. Which of the following is correct regarding this patient's diagnosis and management?

A. Tissue evacuated from the uterine cavity is likely to have a 46,XX karyotype.

B. Treatment should be expectant management.

C. Treatment should be hysterectomy.

D. Treatment should be immediate single agent chemotherapy.

E. There is a 25% risk of recurrence with subsequent pregnancies.

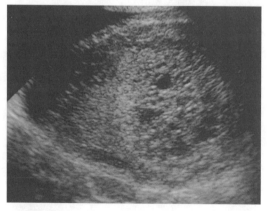

FIGURE 97

QUESTION 98

A 62-year-old G3P3 woman presents to the ED 5 days after undergoing a laparoscopic Burch culposuspension procedure for stress urinary incontinence. She reports that she has only been able to micturate small volumes over the past 6 hr despite constant urgency. Additionally, she is experiencing mild nausea and increasing midline lower abdominal pain without radiation, but denies vomiting, fever, chills, constipation, or loose stools. Her past medical history is noncontributory. Vital signs are within normal limits. On physical exam, you note mild suprapubic pain, normal bowel sounds, and no peritoneal signs. Pelvic exam reveals discomfort with uterine manipulation, but no cervical motion tenderness, vaginal discharge or bleeding, and no uterine, cervical, or adnexal masses. Rectal exam is nontender with normal tone. You collect a 20-cc urine specimen that reveals the following on urine dipstick: specific gravity 1.010, no red blood cells, negative leukocyte esterase, 2–5 bacteria per high power field, and 1–3 squamous cells per high power field. The most appropriate next step in management of this patient is

A. Outpatient treatment of urinary tract infection (UTI)

B. Hospitalization for IV antibiotic treatment

C. Straight catheterization to obtain a clean sample for urinalysis

D. Placement of a Foley catheter

E. Surgical exploration/repair

QUESTION 99

A 31-year-old G1P0 at $38^5/_7$ weeks GA with previously normal blood pressures reports to the ED after home blood pressure monitoring reveals a BP of 148/94. She reports the prenatal course has been uncomplicated. Repeat blood pressure on arrival to the ED is 140/92 and the patient's urine dips 2+ proteinuria. Fetal heart rate (FHR) monitoring is reassuring. You draw the appropriate preeclamptic labs, and as you await their return, the nurse informs you that the patient is having a seizure. Upon your arrival to the bedside, the patient is confused, but no longer seizing. Physical exam is within normal limits, and the lab results are still pending. The FHR tracing reveals a baseline heart rate in the 130s and exhibits decreased variability during the seizure that has since recovered to its prior state of moderate variability. Which of the following is the best management at this point?

A. Administer phenytoin

B. Administer diazepam

C. Administer phenobarbital

D. Administer magnesium sulfate

E. Expectant management

QUESTION 100

A 17-year-old G0 woman with a history of dysmenorrhea and menorrhagia presents to the ED complaining of gradual onset lower abdominal pain and heavy vaginal bleeding that has soaked 5 pads over the past 12 hr. The patient is not sexually active. Her vital signs are stable, and she is afebrile. Physical exam reveals normal bowel sounds and mild lower abdominal tenderness to palpation, but no peritoneal signs or palpable masses. On pelvic exam, you note a small amount of blood in the vaginal vault, but no evidence of active bleeding and no cervical motion tenderness or adnexal masses. Her hematocrit is 31. In addition to starting iron supplementation, which of the following would be appropriate management of this patient?

A. Dilatation and curettage (D&C)

B. Cyclic oral contraceptives (OCPs)

C. GnRH therapy

D. Endometrial ablation

E. Progestin trial (Depo-Provera)

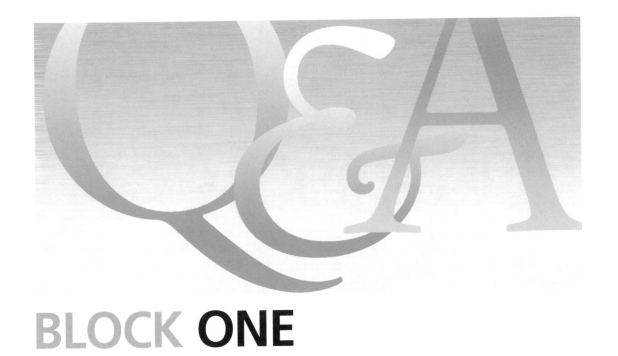

BLOCK **ONE**

ANSWERS

ANSWER 1

A. Roughly 5% of all pregnancies are complicated by asymptomatic bacteriuria of >100,000 colonies on culture, which is similar to the rate seen in the nonpregnant population. However, asymptomatic bacteriuria in pregnant women progresses more frequently to urinary tract infection (UTI), cystitis, and pyelonephritis, as seen in 25% of patients. In 15% of pregnant patients with pyelonephritis, complications may be more severe and include bacteremia, sepsis, and adult respiratory distress syndrome (ARDS). The increased incidence of cystitis and pyelonephritis in pregnancy is due to increased stasis and reflux. The elevated progesterone in pregnancy relaxes smooth muscle which causes decreased bladder tone, ureteral dilation, and decreased ureteral peristalsis. In addition, the mechanical obstruction of the uterus on the bladder and the ureters can result in stasis. Because asymptomatic bacteriuria can progress to severe infection in the pregnant patient, it should be evaluated further, in this case with a urine culture.

B. Following a pregnant woman for symptoms of UTI is somewhat nonspecific. Increased blood flow to the bladder and pressure from the uterus cause most pregnant women to experience frequency and sometimes urgency. Some pregnant women with pyelonephritis will not have experienced symptoms of urinary tract infection.

C. Vaginal flora and discharge may explain the urine dip results. Treating all patients presumptively with antibiotics can lead to increased microbial resistance, allergic reactions, and maternal side effects. Patients with a history of pyelonephritis, urologic surgery, or frequent UTIs may require suppressive treatment during pregnancy.

D. To ignore a urine dip suggestive of a urinary tract infection might result in progression of asymptomatic bacteriuria, putting the patient at risk for pyelonephritis.

E. A renal biopsy is extreme and unnecessary.

ANSWER 2

D. In addition to breast enlargement, the patient has a secondary mound caused by projection of the areola and papilla. This is characteristic of Tanner stage 4. In addition, her pubic hair appears mid-escutcheon, characteristic of Tanner stage 4. The patient's exam suggests the presence of circulating estrogens, as well as normal anatomy, both of which are important in the evaluation of primary amenorrhea.

A. Pre-adolescent breasts, with elevation of the papilla only, and absent pubic hair characterize Tanner stage 1.

B. Breast buds characterize Tanner stage 2. The breast and papilla are elevated, and the areola is engorged. Presexual axillary and pubic hair may be present.

C. Tanner stage 3 is characterized by further development of breast size, without separation in contour from the breast and the areola. Axillary and sexual pubic hair may be present.

E. Tanner stage 5 is the mature stage. The breasts have an adult contour, with recession of the areola. Axillary hair and a female escutcheon are present.

ANSWER 3

D. The most common cause of secondary amenorrhea is pregnancy, which is ruled out in this patient with a negative urine pregnancy test. The patient is extremely thin and should be evaluated for anorexia nervosa. Weight loss, anorexia nervosa, stress, and exercise can all cause hypothalamic dysfunction and disruption in the pulsatile secretion of GnRH, resulting in hypogonadotropic hypogonadism. Most adolescents experience some degree of hypothalamic amenorrhea during the first couple of years after menarche.

A. Cervical stenosis can cause secondary amenorrhea and is usually caused by scarring of the cervical os as a result of obstetric trauma or surgery, both of which this patient denies.

B. Asherman's syndrome, the presence of intrauterine synechiae or adhesions, can cause secondary amenorrhea, but is unlikely in this patient with no history of the usual etiologies, which include infection, intrauterine surgery, and less often, dilation and curettage, cesarean section, myomectomy, and endometritis.

C. Premature ovarian failure (POF) is defined by menopause that occurs before age 40. Chromosomal analysis is sent before the age of 35 to rule out a genetic basis for POF. It may result from radiation, chemotherapy, infection, or ovarian surgery, but is most often idiopathic. While POF is a possible etiology of secondary amenorrhea, the patient has no other symptoms of menopause, making the diagnosis of POF unlikely.

E. Polycystic ovarian disease, originally described as Stein–Leventhal syndrome, represents a spectrum of disease characterized by oligomenorrhea and some degree of chemical or clinical androgenization. These patients are also generally obese. While this is a possible diagnosis, the patient has no evidence of androgenization.

ANSWER 4

B. It is estimated that approximately one-third of women are smokers at the time of conception. Of these women, only approximately 20% are able to quit by the time of their first prenatal visit. Studies have shown that smoking cessation programs, including inquiry and encouragement by health care providers, are quite effective. In fact, smoking cessation programs appear to be more effective during pregnancy. Therefore, it is essential that health care providers inquire about and counsel all patients regarding smoking cessation during pregnancy.

A. Infants of women who smoked during pregnancy have a higher incidence of SIDS and respiratory illnesses during childhood.

C. A clear dose-response relationship correlating smoking with increased harm has been demonstrated. A reduction in the amount smoked, even during pregnancy, is beneficial.

D. Smoking during pregnancy is associated with spontaneous abortion, abruption, and decreased birthweight.

E. See answer B.

ANSWER 5

D. Vertical transmission of HIV occurs from the transplacental route, during birth, and via breast milk. In the first-world, where other sources of infant nutrition are available, breast-feeding is absolutely contraindicated. The patient needs to be made aware of the risk breast-feeding poses to her newborn.

A. Given her absence of other risk factors, there is a significant likelihood that the patient contracted HIV from her husband. He should be screened and, if positive, evaluated for possible anti-retroviral therapy.

B. Various anti-retroviral regimens have shown promise for the reduction of HIV infection. However, currently there is no known cure for HIV.

C. Untreated, approximately 25% of infants born to HIV-infected mothers will become infected. Seventy to 80% of perinatal transmission occurs intrapartum, and the remaining 20–30% is transplacental. Treatment with zidovudine (AZT) was shown to decrease perinatal transmission to 8%. Recent studies have demonstrated further decreases in perinatal transmission with scheduled cesarean section and lower maternal viral load.

E. Patients with higher viral loads and more advanced disease are at greater risk for vertical transmission.

ANSWER 6

C. African American preterm infants actually have lower rates of respiratory distress syndrome when compared to Caucasian infants born at the same gestational ages (GAs). This is also true of female infants when compared to male infants.

A & B. Perinatal morbidity and mortality are significantly higher among African Americans when compared to Caucasians in the United States. One etiology for this is higher rates of prematurity. However, this difference remains even when GA, birthweight, and socioeconomic status are controlled in multivariate analyses.

D. Pregnant women who are African American are more likely to present for prenatal care beyond 12 weeks of gestation than Caucasian women.

E. The incidence of preterm labor and delivery, and preterm rupture of membranes, is significantly higher among African Americans when compared to Caucasians.

ANSWER 7

E. The patient has clear signs of chorioamnionitis, an infection of the chorionic and amniotic membranes as well as the amniotic fluid. The signs and symptoms commonly associated with chorioamnionitis are maternal fever, fetal tachycardia, tender uterus, malodorous vaginal discharge, and maternal leukocytosis; four out of five of these findings makes the diagnosis. Chorioamnionitis is the most common cause of neonatal sepsis, which poses a significant risk for neonatal death. Given the signs and the risks, and despite the early GA, induction of labor should be initiated. The patient should also be treated with intravenous fluids, Tylenol, and broad-spectrum antibiotics that include coverage for group B streptococcus.

A. Cesarean section in this setting should be reserved for a persistently nonreassuring fetal heart tracing, malpresentation, or failed induction. A cesarean section in the setting of chorioamnionitis is associated with increased postpartum complications such as wound infection, abscess, and fistula formation.

B. The patient should receive antibiotics, but observation in the setting of diagnosed chorioamnionitis is inappropriate.

C. Amniocentesis for culture is performed sometimes when the diagnosis is unclear. In this case, the patient clearly has chorioamnionitis. Amniocentesis for culture would only waste critical time.

D. The tampon dye test involves the placement of a tampon in the vagina and injection of indigo carmine into the amniotic cavity; the tampon is removed 1 hr later. Blue die on the tampon confirms rupture of membranes. In this patient's case, the diagnosis of rupture of membranes has been made by history and the findings of ferning, nitrazine positive fluid, and oligohydramnios.

ANSWER 8

A. Metronidazole (Flagyl), dosed orally at 2 g once, is often sufficient treatment for *Trichomonas vaginalis,* the sexually transmitted infection from which this patient suffers. Actively moving, flagellated organisms seen on wet prep in the setting of this patient's symptoms are diagnostic of *Trichomonas.*

B. Partners must always be treated, or they will continue to transmit the infection.

C. The only alternative treatment to Flagyl for *Trichomonas* is clotrimazole vaginal suppositories, used very uncommonly.

D. If a patient is diagnosed with an STD, she is at risk for other STDs and needs full STD screening.

E. Diagnosis can be made on wet prep alone. Therefore, culture is unnecessary to make the diagnosis and may result in delayed treatment or lost treatment opportunity.

ANSWER 9

C. Cervical cerclage is used in the setting of incompetent cervix. This can be either for patients with a history of incompetent cervix in a prior pregnancy or to intervene in an ongoing pregnancy that is threatened by a changing cervix without contractions. This patient does not have the diagnosis of incompetent cervix. Furthermore, cervical cerclage is not advisable in the setting of ruptured membranes, given the high risk of preterm labor and chorioamnionitis.

A. Expectant management at home is unlikely to change the outcome, and probably far less than 10% of previable fetuses with ruptured membranes actually make it to viability. However, after an ultrasound to assess the amniotic fluid and counseling from the obstetrician, many patients may elect expectant management. As long as they are reliable, this is a reasonable approach to care. It is imperative that the patient return in 1 week for reassessment, and sooner if she has temperatures >100.4°F (38°C) or uterine tenderness.

B. Given the potentially grim outcome for this pregnancy, the patient may elect to undergo dilation and evacuation. However, the patient should first be counseled by her obstetrician and then possibly by a neonatologist.

D. One finding that is associated with even worse outcomes is absence of amniotic fluid as noted by ultrasound. That is, those patients who have mid-trimester rupture of the membranes and have normal amniotic fluid have better outcomes than those patients with no amniotic fluid. Thus, an ultrasound to determine this will help in counseling these patients.

E. Given the patient's clear diagnosis of rupture of membranes, she is at high risk for preterm delivery. While many patients elect for expectant management at home, further observation in the hospital overnight or for a few days is not unreasonable. Once the initial 24 hr has passed and there is no evidence of chorioamnionitis, the patient is then discharged for follow-up in a week.

ANSWER 10

B. This patient's multiparity and pregnancy put her at risk for urinary incontinence, which may be the source for her "wetness." However, because some patients may rupture membranes with only a high leak rather than a gush of fluid, a sterile speculum exam should be performed to evaluate for pooling of amniotic fluid in the vagina, which may not always be evident in cases of slow leaks. A sample of vaginal fluid should also be tested for ferning, which occurs because amniotic fluid contains a high concentration of sodium that crystallizes upon drying, forming the characteristic "ferning" pattern observed under microscopy. Amniotic fluid is basic and should turn pH paper blue, which is indicative of a positive nitrazine paper test. If all tests are negative in the setting of high suspicion for ruptured membranes, an ultrasound should be performed to check the amniotic fluid index. In some causes, a tampon dye test may be performed.

A. One must maintain a high index of suspicion for ruptured membranes. Observation at home, when rupture of membranes is suggested by history, is inappropriate.

C. Evaluation for rupture of membranes is of primary importance in this patient. However, the patient should also be checked with a wet prep to rule out BV (bacterial vaginosis) or yeast, as either could explain her symptoms.

D. A GBS (group B streptoccus) culture may be performed in some institutions. Typically, the culture is sent after 24 weeks in patients at risk for preterm delivery.

E. Ultrasound is sometimes performed if suspicion for rupture of membranes is high but the exam is normal. The first test performed, however, should be a sterile speculum exam, to assess for leakage of fluid.

ANSWER 11

B. IV cefoxitin with oral doxycycline is appropriate treatment for PID. However, this patient's signs and symptoms, particularly mucopurulent discharge from the os, cervical-motion tenderness, and sexual history, strongly suggest cervicitis, likely caused by *Neisseria gonorrhoeae* or *Chlamydia trachomatis*. Abdominal pain, adnexal pain, and cervical motion tenderness are the three major criteria for PID. The patient should undergo cervical cultures and receive presumptive treatment. Her partner also needs treatment. Because infection by the two organisms may be clinically indistinguishable, treatment regimens for both cervicitis and PID should cover both organisms. This patient should also be counseled to use condoms for their relative protection against sexually transmitted diseases (STDs) and should be offered full STD-screening, including an HIV test. Among sexually active women, 20- to 24-year-olds have the highest prevalence of gonococcal and chlamydial infections. If left untreated, cervicitis caused by these organisms may progress to PID.

A. This is a common treatment regimen for gonococcal or chlamydial cervicitis, or an outpatient regimen for PID. Ceftriaxone covers *Neisseria gonorrhoeae* (GC) and doxycycline covers *Chlamydia trachomatis* (CT). Patients in whom PID is suspected are often treated in-house due to the high failure rate of outpatient treatment, and possible sequelae of infertility, peritoneal abscess, and chronic PID. Patients who are noncompliant, especially teenagers, those unable to tolerate oral medication, pregnant women, or severely ill patients, require inpatient management.

C. Ofloxacillin may be used to treat cervicitis. GC is covered by 400 mg × 1. To cover chlamydia, however, it needs to be given BID for a week. Thus, the one time dose of azithromycin is often given instead.

D. Two grams of azithromycin has been shown to treat both GC and CT.

E. Ceftriaxone and azithromycin has been the most common way to treat cervicitis.

ANSWER 12

E. In actual use, the failure rate of the oral contraceptive pill is approximately 3%. Patients should be informed that maximum effectiveness of the pill can only be achieved by taking the pill at roughly the same time each day. Additionally, patients should be given instructions for missed doses. If they forget one dose, they should take it as soon as possible and take the following pill at the regularly scheduled time in addition to using a backup method of contraception. If they forget to take the pill for two days, they should take two pills immediately, then take two pills at the next scheduled dose, and then continue to take one pill a day as usual, but use a backup method for the remainder of the package. Missing three or more pills requires that the patient discard the package and start with a new one, using a backup method for the duration of the package.

A. With proper use, the condom can be 98% effective in preventing pregnancy. It is also effective in reducing the transmission of STDs. In actual use, the condom's failure rate is approximately 12%. Patients should be instructed to leave a well at the tip of the condom to collect ejaculate and to avoid leakage of semen when the penis is withdrawn.

B. When no method of contraception is used, the pregnancy rate within 1 year among sexually active women is approximately 85%.

C. The copper T IUD is highly effective and reversible. The IUD is good for women who are monogamous and at low risk for STDs.

D. Vasectomy is simple, safe, and highly effective. Vasectomy involves ligation of the vas deferens and may be performed in the physician's office under local anesthesia.

ANSWER 13

A. The heroin withdrawal syndrome may be more dangerous to the developing fetus than heroin itself. Pregnancy-related side effects of heroin withdrawal include miscarriage, preterm delivery, and fetal death. Methadone is a narcotic commonly used to help wean from heroin use. Changing from heroin to methadone, as long as the methadone dose is adequate, is less harmful to the fetus than is withdrawal from all narcotics.

B. Despite the fact that this patient is presenting for her initial prenatal appointment at 31 weeks GA, all the labs normally obtained in the first trimester are still applicable. These include a rubella titer, RPR, hepatitis B surface antigen, Pap smear, CBC, urinalysis, culture, and increasingly a VZV titer. It is too late to obtain a MSAFP, normally performed between 15 and 20 weeks, to screen for neural tube defects or aneuploidy.

C. As stated above, the fetus and the patient are better off if the patient begins methadone. The infant will need careful monitoring and slow withdrawal from the narcotic after birth. Once the patient delivers, she should undergo aggressive efforts to taper methadone.

D. Given the uncertainty of her dating and significant potential for noncompliance, the patient should undergo ultrasound today for dating and to screen for anomalies.

E. IV drug abuse places the patient at significant risk for HIV. Identification of her status is important, as drugs such as AZT are now used to reduce the risk of vertical transmission. Further, if the patient is HIV positive and her viral load is greater than 1000 copies, she should be offered a cesarean section at term to further reduce the risk of vertical transmission.

ANSWER 14

E. Chicken pox during pregnancy can be quite severe. If a pregnant woman develops vari-cella pneumonia, she is at significant risk of death. This patient is within 72 hr of the time of exposure, so she may benefit from VZIG. Because 70–90% of patients who do not recall having had chicken pox exposure actually have detectable antibodies, and thus do not need VZIG, rapid VZV screening for prior exposure should be performed prior to administration of VZIG.

A. The patient should be told specifically not to come to the clinic, where she could potentially infect other pregnant women.

B. See answer E.

C. Oral acyclovir may reduce the duration of new lesion formation and the total number of lesions if instituted within 24 hr of the rash. Oral acyclovir is safe in pregnancy (class B) and may provide symptomatic relief. It does not, however, reduce the risk of vertical transmission. This patient has no symptoms of varicella, and needs further evaluation before you prescribe medication.

D. VZIG should be given to infants born to women who develop varicella between 5 days prior to and 2 days after delivery. If this patient develops varicella and delivers within 5 days, the pediatrician needs to be alerted and the infant prophylaxed.

ANSWER 15

D. The incidence of invasive cervical cancer is substantially higher among HIV-infected women. In fact, invasive cervical cancer has been categorized as an AIDS-defining illness. Given the increased incidence, HIV-infected women must undergo at least annual Pap smear surveillance, possibly more frequently depending upon personal history.

A. The CDC recommends that HIV-infected women undergo a repeat Pap smear in 6 months. If the initial and the repeat are both normal, and the patient does not have AIDS or is without a history of HPV, squamous intraepithelial neoplasia, or symptomatic HIV, the Pap smear may be repeated annu-ally. Otherwise, she should have a Pap smear every 6 months.

B. See answer D.

C. See answer A.

E. HIV works synergistically with HPV, leading to more frequent invasive disease in women with both.

ANSWER 16

D. Uterine fibroids are the sole cause of infertility in 2–10% of cases. Fibroid-related infertility may be due to distortion of the endocervical canal, endometrial cavity, or fallopian tubes, interfering with conception or implantation, and sometimes causing spontaneous abortion.

A. An estimated 20–30% of American women develop fibroids by age 40, and 50–65% have no clinical symptoms. The most common symptom is abnormal vaginal bleeding, as seen in this patient. Pressure-related symptoms are relatively common. Symptoms generally depend on the location of the fibroids, as evidenced in this patient, with the posterior location of her fairly large fibroid causing dyspareunia and constipation.

B. Studies suggest that the degeneration of a fibroid to a leiomyosarcoma occurs rarely (approximately 1:1000). Rapidly enlarging fibroids in a postmenopausal woman or uncertain diagnosis are causes for concern, but possible malignant potential is not a typical indication for fibroid removal.

C. Estrogen stimulates fibroid growth, causing some fibroids to increase significantly during pregnancy and to regress after menopause. Fibroid growth during pregnancy may lead to problems such as severe pain due to infarction as a fibroid outgrows its blood supply. Other problems include intrauterine growth restriction (IUGR), uterine distortion causing malpresentation, preterm labor, and dystocia (blockage of the presenting part necessitating a cesarean section).

E. African American women have three to nine times the incidence of uterine fibroids when compared to Hispanic, Asian, and Caucasian women.

ANSWER 17

C. Because congenital syphilis can be quite severe and treatment for syphilis is available, syphilis is screened for universally in pregnancy by the rapid plasmin reagin (RPR) test. Since the RPR is a nonspecific screening test and carries a high false-positive rate, diagnosis should be confirmed with the more specific microhemagglutination assay for antibodies to *Treponema pallidum* (MHA-TP) or the fluorescent treponemal antibody-absorption (FTA-ABS) technique before any action is taken.

A & B. Patients with rheumatologic disease have a higher incidence of false-positive screening for syphilis and are sometimes identified this way. However, this patient has no symptoms of lupus or rheumatoid arthritis. Her history of fatigue is quite mild and nonspecific. Given her lack of symptoms of rheumatologic disease, sending an ANA, which also carries a high false-positive rate, is not indicated. Further evaluation for syphilis is the most appropriate next step.

D. Early syphilis is treated with penicillin G 2.4 million units IM once. Confirmatory testing is needed prior to treatment, with the possible exception of a highly noncompliant patient at high-risk for syphilis (e.g., known positive partner).

E. Rather than repeat a nonspecific test, one should send the more specific confirmatory test.

ANSWER 18

D. CIN III, or severe dysplasia, is described as high-grade SIL (HGSIL) and is likely to progress to cervical cancer if left untreated. Excision of the lesion is necessary. The endocervical curettage was performed to assess the endocervical canal, which cannot be viewed during colposcopy. This patient has no abnormal tissue identified by endocervical curettage. However, because one of the lesions appears to extend into the canal, it is imperative to excise the endocervical canal. This can be done in the office with a LEEP or in the OR with a cold knife cone biopsy.

A. HPV is the primary cause of cervical cancer and premalignant lesions. Serotypes 16, 18, and 31 are especially correlated with cervical cancer. Serotyping for HPV can be used to guide management in cases of atypical squamous cells of undetermined significance (ASCUS). Some clinicians will use serotyping to determine who should be evaluated by immediate colposcopy versus repeat Pap smear and HPV serotyping in 6 months. However, it is not useful in cases of more advanced lesions, such as this patient's, where excision is indicated.

B & C. In this setting, it is important to obtain tissue for a diagnosis as well as ensure removal of the endocervical lesion, confirm negative margins, and evaluate for focal sites of cervical carcinoma within the HGSIL. Cryotherapy and laser ablation both destroy the tissue, preventing the assessment of margins. Furthermore, although the patient does not have endocervical abnormalities, neither method is particularly useful for treating endocervical lesions.

E. Patients with ASCUS and CIN I may be followed with colposcopy every 3–4 months. If left untreated, approximately 30% of CIN I lesions will resolve. It takes about 7 years for CIN I lesions to progress to cervical cancer. However, patients with HGSIL (CIN II and CIN III) should be treated aggressively.

ANSWER 19

A. The diaphragm should be left in place for 6–8 hr after intercourse; removal sooner may result in pregnancy. The annual failure rate for the diaphragm with spermicide is 18% despite a theoretical failure rate of 6%, largely because of misuse.

B. Patients should be counseled that additional spermicide should be used for each subsequent act of intercourse prior to diaphragm removal.

C. Poor diaphragm fit caused by old material or body changes (a weight change of greater than 10 lb) may lead to diaphragm failure. The diaphragm is held in place by its fit in the vaginal canal, which may change in size with alterations in weight. Regardless, the diaphragm should be replaced every 5 years.

D. As with tampons, colonization with *Staphylococcus aureus* may lead to toxic shock syndrome if the diaphragm is left in place for too long.

E. See answer A.

ANSWER 20

A. Germ cell tumors include teratomas, dysgerminomas, endodermal sinus tumors, and choriocarcinoma. Classification of ovarian neoplasms is based upon the cell of origin: surface epithelial, germ, and sex-cord stromal cells. Epithelial cell neoplasms are the most common, and mucinous and endometrioid tumors arise from this group.

B. Epithelial cell tumors are the most common and give rise to benign and malignant tumors. Major categories of epithelial tumors include serous and mucinous tumors, endometrioid clear cell, undifferentiated carcinoma, and the Brenner tumor.

C. The major types of sex-cord stromal tumors include Granulosa-theca and Sertoli-Leydig cell tumors as well as gonadoblastomas.

D. While epithelial cell tumors affect women age 20 and older, they are most frequent among women in their late 50s.

E. Germ cell tumors generally affect girls and women of 0–25 years of age. As with all tumors, they may be seen at any age.

ANSWER 21

B. The prevalence of domestic violence during pregnancy appears to increase, ranging from 1–20% with most studies reporting rates between 4% and 8%. A current or prior intimate partner is usually the perpetrator. While risks for domestic violence, such as partner control or multiple somatic complaints, are sometimes apparent, this is often not the case. Thus, universal screening should be employed. Examples of screening questions include:

i. Has anyone close to you ever threatened to hurt you?

ii. Have you ever been afraid of your partner?

iii. Has anyone ever hit, kicked, choked, or hurt you physically?

iv. Has anyone, including your partner, ever forced you to have sex?

A. The biophysical profile is used most frequently to follow up a nonreactive NST. It involves evaluation of the following variables: fetal breathing movements, fetal tone, fetal heart rate reactivity, fetal movements, and qualitative amniotic fluid volume.

C. Although supportive inquiry regarding the patient's lack of weight gain might be beneficial, her concern regarding this issue makes the diagnosis of anorexia nervosa unlikely.

D & E. There is no indication for ultrasound or weekly non-stress tests at this point.

ANSWER 22

D. This patient has evidence of placental abruption, which is highly associated with cocaine use during pregnancy, making cocaine the most likely substance found on urine tox screen. The mechanisms for abruption are unclear but include elevated blood pressures, vasospasm in the placental bed, and uterotonic effects. Cocaine is also associated with preterm delivery, intrauterine growth restriction (IUGR), and developmental delay in neonates.

A. Marijuana has not been associated with any particular adverse perinatal outcomes.

B. Ethyl alcohol (EtOH) has been associated with fetal alcohol syndrome (FAS). This syndrome involves a constellation of findings including IUGR, CNS effects, abnormal facies, and frequent cardiac anomalies. While there certainly appears to be a dose-response effect, it is unclear if there is a safe level of alcohol consumption in pregnancy.

C. Benzodiazepine abuse in pregnancy has also been associated with several cases of a syndrome that resembles FAS.

E. While opiates have not been shown to be particularly teratogenic in pregnancy, they have been associated with preterm delivery and fetal death.

ANSWER 23

B. Dysgerminoma, a germ cell tumor of the ovary predominantly affecting girls and young women, is remarkable for its secretion of LDH as a tumor marker. Germ cell tumors of the ovary arise from totipotential cells. Patients commonly present with a rapidly enlarging adnexal mass and abdominal pain.

A. Choriocarcinoma is a germ cell tumor and also a form of gestational trophoblastic disease that secretes HCG.

C. Embryonal carcinomas may produce HCG, AFP, as well as CA-125.

D. Endodermal sinus tumors may produce AFP.

E. Immature teratomas or immature dermoid cysts may produce CA-125.

ANSWER 24

B. A complex ovarian mass in a post-menopausal woman requires a diagnostic and staging laparotomy. The patient's signs and symptoms, in particular the complex mass in the setting of ascites, are particularly concerning for ovarian cancer. Exploratory laparotomy is performed to make a diagnosis and, if cancer is found, to debulk the tumor.

A. The postmenopausal ovary does not cycle. A complex ovarian cyst in a post-menopausal woman is highly suspicious for carcinoma and is not expected to resolve. A delay in diagnosis is potentially harmful.

C. Diuretic treatment of ascites has little efficacy, as fluid reaccumulates. As fluid returns to the third-space, the patient may become intravascularly depleted and dehydrated. Thus, diuretic treatment of ascites can be harmful.

D. A second opinion is reserved for cases in which management is unclear or controversial, which is not the case here. A patient may always seek a second opinion herself, a decision that should be supported.

E. If ovarian carcinoma is found, the patient will undergo surgical debulking of her tumor followed by chemotherapy. Until an accurate tissue diagnosis is made, chemotherapy should not be performed. Debulking the tumor is also thought to increase the percentage of tumor in S-phase, making the tumor relatively more responsive to chemotherapy than the patient's normal tissue.

ANSWER 25

E. The patient described above has signs and symptoms consistent with polycystic ovarian disease (PCOD). However, since the leading cause of secondary amenorrhea in reproductive aged women is pregnancy, the patient should be evaluated with a urine pregnancy test. It is important to remember that what a patient describes as a light period may actually be spotting during pregnancy. Once pregnancy is ruled out, other causes of amenorrhea may be sought.

A. The patient has clinical signs of androgenization. She is described as hirsute, which suggests an elevated testosterone. While not critical to making the diagnosis of PCOD, given the patient's appearance, one could order a free serum testosterone to confirm chemical hyperandrogenism. Oligomenorrhea in the setting of androgenization suggests PCOD.

B & C. Both thyroid dysfunction and prolactinoma may cause irregular menses and should be included in the workup.

D. Insulin resistance and hyperinsulinemia are common in patients with PCOD who are obese and hyperandrogenic. This patient needs screening for type II diabetes, which is increased in these patients. Weight loss should be discussed with the patient. Even modest weight loss can increase her ovulation and would reduce her risk of type II diabetes.

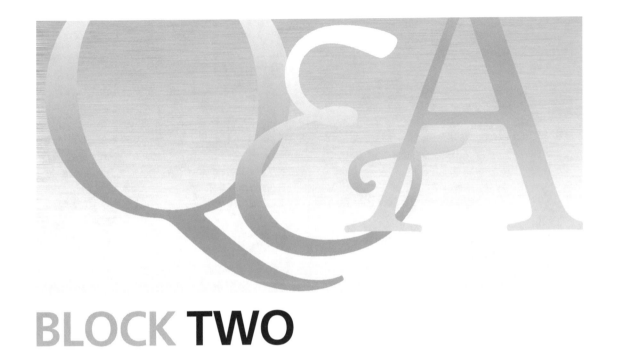

BLOCK TWO

ANSWERS

ANSWER 26

B. First trimester ultrasound utilizing mean sac diameter or crown-rump length is the most consistent way to date a pregnancy. In general, first trimester ultrasound is considered to be within 4–7 days of accurate dating. Thus, if the dating by LMP is off by a week or more in the first trimester, dating should be reconsidered and be based upon the ultrasound.

A. LMP can be quite accurate, particularly in a patient with a certain LMP and regular menstrual cycles. However, this form of dating needs to be substantiated by ultrasound because irregular menses, poor documentation of the LMP, and ovulation other than on Day 14 of the cycle can lead to poor dating.

C. Second-trimester ultrasound uses biometry of the biparietal diameter, head circumference, abdominal circumference, and femur length to help determine dating. Generally, this form of dating is felt to be within 7–14 days.

D. The third-trimester ultrasound is a notoriously inaccurate form of dating. Estimates of the EDC can be off by as much as 3 weeks.

E. While beta-HCG values have been used to determine whether a pregnancy is normal, they are not well associated with exact dating of gestational age (GA).

ANSWER 27

E. With the increasing availability of medical options for pregnancy termination, including the recently approved mifepristone (RU-486, Mifeprex), it is likely that these interventions will be increasingly practiced by gynecologists as well as family practice physicians. However, high-dose estrogen and progesterone pills are used for emergency contraception, also known as the morning-after pill, rather than for medical abortion. Traditionally given as high-dose OCPs, emergency contraception is now available as a separate medication, often in combination with a urine pregnancy test. It is given in two doses, 12 hr apart, and should be used within 72 hr of unprotected intercourse.

A. Mifepristone (RU-486) has received an enormous amount of press over the past decade. Its method of action is via binding of progesterone receptors in the endometrium, which is then thought to interrupt the pregnancy. When given alone, it is 80–85% effective. This efficacy increases to >90% when given with a prostaglandin such as misoprostol.

B. Misoprostol, a prostaglandin—PGE1M, can be used alone as a first-trimester abortifacient with an efficacy ranging 50–90%. It is often used in conjunction with either methotrexate or mifepristone to increase the combined efficacy to over 90%.

C. See answer B.

D. See answer A.

ANSWER 28

A. Infertility is classically defined as 12 months or more of unprotected intercourse not resulting in a pregnancy. This couple has only been trying for 9 months. Given her age of 39, however, it is important to assess the situation and intervene quickly because of the decreasing probability of pregnancy with advancing maternal age. In this patient with irregular menses, it is likely that she is anovulatory or oligo-ovulatory (only a few ovulatory cycles per year). Assessing whether she is ovulating is important and can be done in a variety of ways. However, the LH/FSH ratio, which was classically used to diagnose polycystic ovarian syndrome, is not one of those ways.

B. The basal body temperature is the least expensive way to verify ovulation and has the benefit of identifying when ovulation occurs for patients attempting to do timed intercourse.

C. If ovulation occurs, the resulting corpus luteum secretes progesterone, which helps the endometrium mature into an environment suitable for implantation. Thus, an elevated progesterone level after Day 21 of the cycle is consistent with ovulation. This method might be more difficult in this patient because of the irregularity in her cycles, but it can still be utilized.

D. Luteinizing hormone (LH) rises in a spike immediately prior to ovulation. Thus, testing for elevated LH levels in the serum or urine is predictive for both the presence and timing of ovulation. Urine LH kits are available over the counter and have become the first-line assessment for ovulation.

E. Just like checking a luteal phase progesterone level, a luteal phase endometrial biopsy allows a histologic view of the hormonal milieu the endometrium is experiencing. Evidence of an appropriate endometrial response to progesterone can be reassuring for the occurrence of ovulation.

ANSWER 29

D. The MSAFP is an important aspect of the prenatal screen in the second trimester. It is used alone to screen for neural tube defects (spina bifida, anencephaly) and in combination with unconjugated estriol and beta-HCG to screen for trisomies 18 and 21. An elevated MSAFP is associated with neural tube defects and both trisomies are associated with a low MSAFP. However, this testing is done between 15 and 19 weeks of gestation, not at the early gestation of this patient.

A. The RPR is used to screen for syphilis. In pregnancy, this is usually performed in the first trimester and again in the third trimester. Patients with syphilis are at risk of infecting their child, leading to congenital syphilis. Screening for syphilis, confirming diagnosis with either the FTA-ABS or MHA-TP tests, and treating with penicillin can markedly reduce the risk to the fetus.

B. A rubella titer is routinely sent during the first trimester. However, if the patient has a negative titer, she will not be immunized until after the pregnancy because of the small risk that receiving the live virus particles may confer during pregnancy.

C. A HepBsAg titer is also sent in the first trimester. If positive, the patient needs to be evaluated for her status with liver function tests (LFTs) and further antibody testing.

E. A complete blood count is a routine part of the prenatal tests, usually done in the first and third trimesters. First-trimester patients with borderline anemia should be further evaluated. An iron deficiency anemia in the third trimester is common and should be treated with iron supplementation.

ANSWER 30

D. Screening for trisomy 18 is via serum screening, of which MSAFP is a part. However, the risk for trisomy 18 (and trisomy 21) is increased with an MSAFP value that is lower than normal, not elevated. Elevations of MSAFP can be seen in cases of neural tube defects (anencephaly, spina bifida), abdominal wall defects (omphalocele, gastroschisis), improper dating of the pregnancy to an earlier than correct gestational age, fetal demise, and multiple gestations. Cases of unexplained MSAFP elevation are associated with higher rates of pregnancy complications and have been attributed to abnormal placental function.

A. In cases of anencephaly, AFP is released from the neural tissue into the amniotic fluid, and subsequently crosses into maternal circulation.

B. Because of the increased number of fetuses, more AFP crosses into the maternal circulation.

C. AFP is primarily made in the fetal neural tissue and liver. Thus any break in the abdominal integument can allow increased levels to be released into the amniotic fluid and subsequently into the maternal circulation.

E. Use of the MSAFP as a screening test is dependent upon accurate dating of the pregnancy. Because MSAFP increases during the second trimester, false-positive tests can occur if a patient is actually several weeks further along in pregnancy than indicated by her dating.

ANSWER 31

A. In addition to fetal sex, examining fetal extremities is not a part of the routine Level I ultrasound, usually performed between 18 and 21 weeks of gestation. A Level I ultrasound usually includes location of pregnancy (i.e., intrauterine vs. ectopic), location of placenta, amniotic fluid assessment, fetal lie, fetal biometric data for dating, and basic fetal anatomy. The anatomy scan routinely identifies cerebral landmarks such as the ventricles, thalamus, cerebellar hemispheres, and posterior fossa, four-chamber view of the heart, stomach, spine, kidneys, bladder, and umbilical cord insertion.

B. One advantage of ultrasound is the ability to identify the number of fetuses, and if performed early enough, their chorionicity.

C. Fetal kidneys are examined on a routine obstetric ultrasound. Of note, renal pelvis dilation has been associated with aneuploidy and urinary obstruction.

D. There are a variety of disorders associated with abnormal amniotic fluid volume. Polyhydramnios (excess fluid) is associated with diabetes and esophageal atresia, whereas oligohydramnios (diminished fluid) is associated with bladder outlet obstruction.

E. Placental location, and in particular its relationship to the internal cervical os (known as placenta previa if the os is covered in any way by the placenta), is important diagnostic information gained from the Level I ultrasound.

ANSWER 32

D. This patient's history and physical are consistent with an abscess. The location is either vulvar, vaginal, or Bartholin's. Bartholin's gland is located generally just beyond the labia minora and in front of the hymeneal ring. Bartholin's cyst abscesses need to be opened and probed extensively when diagnosed, taking care to make sure that patients realize they need to be followed for several weeks until symptoms resolve. Often, Bartholin's cyst abscesses are not opened up entirely, but are instead treated by creation of a tract into the abscess and placement of a Word catheter, which fits inside the neck of the abscess and is inflated with water once inside. A small amount of fluid is then withdrawn each week until the cyst closes entirely. Recurrent Bartholin cyst abscesses can be incised, drained, and marsupialized. See Figure 32B.

A. Vulvar abscesses would be outside of the vagina and are more common in diabetic and immunosuppressed patients.

B. A vaginal abscess is also a possibility; however, the location is incorrect.

C. Herpes labialis may present with a prodrome of elevated temperatures and inguinal lymphadenopathy. However, it is unusual to present without any vesicular lesions and is not associated with a mass.

E. Condyloma can be seen in many settings. However, their appearance is quite different from the description here.

ANSWER 33

B. Antepartum testing that is performed beyond $40^1/_2$ to 41 weeks gestation in pregnancy is called post-dates testing. Patients with reassuring testing have been shown to have lower rates of IUFD fetuses as compared to high-risk patients without testing. Options for testing include the following: non-stress test (NST), contraction stress test (CST), modified biophysical profile (BPP) (NST plus amniotic fluid assessment), and a complete BPP (evaluation of five diagnostic criteria including fetal tone, movement, breathing motion along with amniotic fluid and an NST). In many high-risk pregnancies, this testing is begun between 32 and 34 weeks of gestation.

A. Gestational diabetes is diagnosed early in the third trimester (if not earlier). It is never tested for in the post-dates period.

C. The likelihood of meconium in the amniotic fluid increases with gestational age. Its most dangerous complication is the risk of meconium aspiration syndrome, which carries a high rate of morbidity for the fetus. However, it cannot be identified by a non-stress test.

D. Macrosomia (a fetus >4000–4500 g by varying definitions) is seen at higher rates in post-dates pregnancies. It is also associated with increased rates of cesarean delivery and shoulder dystocia at birth. Again, this cannot be identified by the non-stress test.

E. Preeclampsia is a syndrome of high blood pressure, proteinuria, and nondependent edema seen in pregnancy. Patients with preeclampsia should undergo early antepartum testing starting at 32–34 weeks of gestation. There is no association between an abnormal non-stress test and development of preeclampsia.

ANSWER 34

C. An Rh-negative mother who is sensitized against anti-D creates IgG antibodies that cross the placenta and can attack fetal erythrocytes leading to fetal hemolytic anemia and eventually high output failure, known as fetal hydrops. We know that the father in this case is Rh positive because he has previously fathered an Rh-positive child with an Rh-negative woman and that he is heterozygous because he also fathered an Rh-negative child. The probability that he will produce an Rh-negative fetus is equal to 0.5. In this case, the numerator is half of the probability of the heterozygotes ($\frac{1}{2} \times 2pq = pq$). The denominator is equal to the probability of having at least one D allele ($2pq$). Thus the overall probability is $pq/(2pq)$. It can also be seen that as we know he is heterozygous, there is a 50% chance that he will pass on the D allele and a 50% chance that he will pass on the – allele. In this case, "-" is used instead of "d" because there is no recessive allele.

A. With no other information, there is a $2pq$ probability of being heterozygous. This equals $2 \times 0.4 \times 0.6 = 0.48$ in Caucasians. However, we know that this patient's husband fathered an Rh-negative person and an Rh-positive person. Thus, the husband is heterozygous.

B. From above, the husband is Rh positive.

D. Rhogam has no use in patients who are already sensitized.

E. As long as the antibody titer remains at 1:8 or lower, there is no reason to perform any amniocenteses. Serial amniocenteses for hemoglobin breakdown products are only necessary at titers of 1:16 or beyond.

ANSWER 35

E. Estrogen (Hormone) replacement therapy (HRT) has been extensively studied and appears to prophylax against both osteoporosis and heart disease in patients at risk for developing these conditions. In addition, HRT can relieve symptoms of hot flashes, mood swings, vaginal dryness, and depression while a patient is transitioning into menopause. HRT does not seem to lower blood pressure or increase the risk of stroke.

A. Hot flashes are among the symptoms that improve with HRT. If a patient declines HRT, they can sometimes get relief with clonidine.

B. When HRT is given in a cyclic fashion, the patient will continue to cycle with regular menses. Over several years, these menses will get lighter until they eventually disappear entirely. At that point, the cyclic HRT is usually changed to continuous.

C. In patients at risk for osteoporosis, estrogen replacement maintains bone density and can prevent osteoporosis.

D. Estrogen affects the lipid profile by increasing HDLs and lowering LDLs, as well as preventing atherogenic plaque development via effects on the endothelium. This combination appears to exert a preventative effect against coronary disease.

ANSWER 36

C. This patient's history is a classic presentation of one of the uterine outflow obstruction syndromes. These include imperforate hymen, transverse vaginal septum, and vaginal agenesis with either a rudimentary uterine horn or entire uterus. When these patients go through menarche, the lack of vaginal egress of menses leads to retrograde menstrual flow into the peritoneal cavity and subsequent cyclic pain. In addition, patients with imperforate hymen and transverse vaginal septum can have a build-up of menses that collects in the upper vagina, which can stretch over time and contain a large volume of old menstrual discharge. In this case, the diagnosis is either imperforate hymen or transverse vaginal septum because of the fullness noted by the patient and clinician. The latter is the more consistent diagnosis because a normal, patent hymeneal ring is noted.

A. Testicular feminization also may present with a foreshortened vagina. Because these patients don't have a uterus; however, the history regarding cyclical pain is inconsistent with testicular feminization.

B. Imperforate hymen is the second most likely diagnosis and often these two are indistinguishable. However, the presence of a clear hymeneal ring near the introitus with vagina beyond confirms the diagnosis of transverse vaginal septum.

D. Labial fusion is seen more commonly in either newborns, young children, or post-menopausal women secondary to a hypoestrogenic state and/or excessive androgenic state.

E. Patients with transverse vaginal septum are most likely to have a normal uterus, tubes, and ovaries.

ANSWER 37

A. Choroid plexus cysts (CPCs) have been associated with both trisomy 21 and trisomy 18 in the reported literature. However, the association with trisomy 21 is tenuous and not generally supported at this time by geneticists. CPCs are associated with trisomy 18, which can then be formally diagnosed by amniocentesis. However, trisomy 18 can be screened for by obstetric ultrasound, which can identify the following associated major structural defects: rocker bottom foot, clubfoot, overriding digits, omphalocele, and cerebral malformations such as holoprosencephaly.

B. The lack of a fetal skull on ultrasound examination is usually how anencephaly is diagnosed. This is the most severe form of the neural tube defects and is not compatible with life.

C. Neural tube defects (NTDs) can be difficult to diagnose by ultrasound, but cerebral findings such as the "lemon" sign (indentation of the frontal bones) and the "banana" sign (obliteration of the posterior fossa by the cerebellar hemispheres that appear to be pulled posteriorly) can help. Most NTDs are found by elevated MSAFP on second trimester serum screening.

D. CPC has not been associated with any long-term poor outcomes in fetuses with normal chromosomes.

E. Turner's syndrome is a sex chromosomal abnormality (45XO) that results in a syndrome of short stature, webbed neck, shield-shaped chest, wide-spaced nipples, and often infertility. These women have relatively normal intelligence. Turner's syndrome has not been associated with CPCs.

ANSWER 38

B. This patient gives an excellent history for endometriosis. It is likely she has endometriotic implants in her pelvis that undergo the same cycle as her endometrium and become inflamed each month with her menses. Over time, these implants can become scarred, cause adhesions, and lead to pain that is intermenstrual and eventually continuous. This pain can become quite debilitating, leading to change in work, school, and social habits. The first step in the treatment of endometriosis is with oral contraceptive pills and nonsteroidal antiinflammatory drugs. If the patient notes relief from pain except during menses, the contraceptive pills can be given continuously with just one or two withdrawal bleeds per year.

A. Laparoscopy in the setting of endometriosis and pelvic pain in general should be used after the patient has failed medical treatment. Laparoscopy is the gold standard for diagnosis of endometriosis, allowing biopsy for pathological confirmation and resection of endometrial implants. Resection of the implants and lysis of adhesions has also been shown to give symptomatic relief. This relief, however, is rarely permanent.

C. Gonadotropin releasing hormone (GnRH) is used in severe cases of endometriosis. It causes ovarian suppression and effectively causes a menopausal-like state. While this can give symptomatic relief, it can also lead to other problems due to prolonged hypoestrogenic state, such as osteoporosis. Any patient undergoing GnRH therapy should have a bone density scan at baseline and have them followed during treatment.

D. Consultation with the pain service and psychiatry service can be an important aspect of management. However, this can often lead to alienation of the patient who may infer that you think her pain is "in her head." Thus, it is better to provide medical therapy first and form a therapeutic bond with the patient. If the medical therapy fails, then you should consider these consults prior to surgery.

E. Although both chronic PID and endometritis are treatable causes of chronic pain, this patient's story is not consistent with either diagnosis. Cultures should be taken at the initial exam to rule PID out.

ANSWER 39

C. While the standard percentiles are made based on Caucasian weights, there is no strong evidence that other ethnicities should have infants that are dramatically different when controlling for factors that do affect birthweight such as fetal sex (F<M), maternal birthweight, gestational age, and multiparity (neonates from subsequent births weigh more on average than those born prior). Factors that are associated with intrauterine growth restriction (IUGR) include longstanding progestational diabetes, chronic hypertension, maternal infections, teratogenic drug exposure, radiation, and chromosomal abnormalities.

A. There are a handful of maternal infections that have been shown to increase pregnancy loss in the first and early second trimester and decrease birthweight later in pregnancy. These include cytomegalovirus, HIV, Rubella, syphilis, VZV, and toxoplasmosis.

B. Many fetuses with chromosomal abnormalities are IUGR.

D. Chronic hypertension and other maternal diseases that lead to vascular disease such as systemic lupus erythematosus (SLE), antiphospholipid antibody syndrome, and longstanding diabetes, lead to poor placental perfusion and IUGR.

E. Maternal birthweight has been the demographic factor most closely associated with fetal birthweight. This association is stronger than paternal birthweight, current maternal and paternal biometrics, and ethnicity.

ANSWER 40

B. Gestational diabetes is a phenomenon seen in pregnancy related to diminished ability to metabolize and utilize carbohydrates efficiently. It is likely a product of a combination of factors including a baseline mild carbohydrate intolerance combined with anti-insulin agents synthesized by the placenta (e.g., human placental lactogen, HPL) that increase throughout the second and third trimesters of pregnancy. Gestational diabetics are divided into two classes: A1 (diet controlled) and A2 (insulin dependent). Gestational diabetes has been associated with increased birthweight and birth injury, but not with fetal anomalies like progestational diabetes. It is also associated with increased likelihood of maternal type II diabetes in the future. Risk factors for developing gestational diabetes include prior gestational diabetes, prior macrosomic fetus, first-degree relative with diabetes, and Latino, South Pacific Islander, or Native American ethnicity.

A. Because the GLT is a screening test and has many false-positive results, an elevated GLT in a prior pregnancy has not been shown to increase risk of diabetes in a subsequent pregnancy.

C. While a history of affected second-degree relatives has not been well studied as a risk factor, it seems likely that there is a mild association with the development of gestational diabetes. However, it is not as strong as the other risk factors listed earlier.

D. The patient did not have gestational diabetes in her last pregnancy; otherwise this would be the strongest risk factor.

E. Prior cesarean section has not been associated with gestational diabetes in epidemiologic studies.

ANSWER 41

E. This patient's syndrome of hirsutism and anovulation along with physical findings of acanthosis nigricans (velvety, thickened skin in the axilla, and nape of the neck) is consistent with polycystic ovarian syndrome (PCOS). Also known as polycystic ovarian disorder (PCOD) or simply PCO, this is a syndromic condition first described by Stein and Leventhal in the setting of hirsutism, virilism, anovulation, amenorrhea, and obesity. It is also associated with insulin resistance and, hence, Type II diabetes. Without any other etiology for her symptoms, this diagnosis can be made. However, an LH/FSH ratio of greater than 3 is also used to confirm this diagnosis of exclusion. But use of this ratio can miss the diagnosis in morbidly obese anovulatory patients who have suppression of their gonadotropins and thus will not have an elevated ratio.

A. Ovarian tumors that can lead to hirsutism and virilism include the sex-cord mesenchymal tumors, granulosa-theca cell tumors, germ cell tumors, and the Sertoli-Leydig cell tumors. These tumors can all secrete testosterone and, hence, a testosterone elevation is often observed. Furthermore, virilism due to ovarian tumors usually presents more acutely with rapid onset of symptoms.

B. Congenital adrenal hyperplasia (CAH) results from a constellation of enzyme deficiencies, the most common being an absence in 21-α-hydroxylase, which results in excess 17-α-hydroxyprogesterone and can lead to the complete inability to synthesize cortisol or mineralocorticoids. Adult-onset CAH can be quite mild with anovulation and androgenization but should still have elevated dehydroepiandrosterone sulfate (DHEA-S) and/or testosterone.

C. Testicular feminization is most commonly related to absence or dysfunction of the testosterone receptor. These patients are genetically 46XY but are phenotypically female. Because of the testosterone receptor dysfunction, they cannot become hirsute or virilized.

D. See answer A.

ANSWER 42

D. Uterine prolapse or vault prolapse in patients who have undergone hysterectomy can be quite uncomfortable and an annoyance to patients. Furthermore, the bladder can be brought down with the prolapse and cause kinking of the bladder neck, requiring vaginal splinting in order to micturate. Risk factors for pelvic relaxation include multiparity, chronic increase in intra-abdominal pressure from cough or ascites, and a hypoestrogenic state. Treatment of prolapse can be medical or surgical. However, the Burch culposuspension procedure is used to restore the bladder neck anatomically in patients with stress incontinence, and would thus be of very little help in this patient's prolapse.

A. Vaginal pessaries are an excellent alternative to surgery. They are placed in the vagina to keep the prolapse from occurring. There are many shapes and sizes, and most women can find one that fits comfortably and provides adequate support for the prolapsing structure.

B. The atrophy secondary to decreased estrogen is a component of prolapse. Thus, oral hormone replacement therapy or topical estrogen cream can help restore some of the strength to the local tissue.

C. Kegel exercises may help strengthen the pelvic floor, which will, in turn, support the pelvic organs.

E. Surgical therapy for vaginal vault or uterine prolapse is usually the abdominal sacrocolpopexy or the vaginal sacrospinous ligament suspension. Colpocleisis, complete closure of the vagina, can be reserved for patients who are poor surgical candidates and no longer desire sexual activity.

ANSWER 43

C. Preeclampsia, except in rare cases of gestational trophoblastic disease such as a molar pregnancy, is almost unheard of prior to 18–20 weeks of pregnancy. In general, it presents in the third trimester, and only severe cases will present in the mid to late second trimester. This patient likely has elevated blood pressure secondary to poor hypertension management.

A. While Aldomet is still commonly used in many patients because it has not been associated with any poor pregnancy outcomes, it is not a particularly effective antihypertensive. This patient was on atenolol at baseline, which could be restarted. However, labetalol gives alpha blockade in addition to beta blockade and is usually the beta-blocker of choice in pregnancy. Another excellent antihypertensive in pregnancy is nifedipine.

B. Because of this patient's increased risk for preeclampsia in the future, assessing baseline LFTs and particularly creatinine is important. A CBC is a routine part of every pregnant patient's prenatal labs.

D. Because this patient has chronic hypertension, it is important to know whether she also has baseline renal dysfunction. This can be done with a 24-hr urine collection for creatinine clearance in conjunction with a serum creatinine.

E. In addition to the creatinine clearance, it is also important to know the baseline protein excretion in order to know both the patient's underlying health state as well as to be able to make the diagnosis of preeclampsia later.

ANSWER 44

B. This patient presents most likely with incompetent cervix, which is silent, painless dilation of the cervix without contractions, usually occurring in the mid to late second trimester. Unfortunately, most diagnoses of incompetent cervix are made when it is too late to intervene to benefit the current pregnancy. Future management is to place a prophylactic cerclage between 12 and 14 weeks of gestation. In this pregnancy, because her cervix is still of reasonable length and only 1 cm dilated, a rescue cerclage can be placed. Because there are no randomized controlled trials for rescue cerclages, which have been associated with infection and rupture of the membranes, expectant management and bed rest is also a reasonable alternative.

A. While bacterial vaginosis (BV) is associated with preterm delivery, this patient does not have BV.

C. There is no particular association of chromosomal abnormalities and incompetent cervix. Furthermore, clinically, this patient is likely at higher risk of complications from amniocentesis than an uncomplicated patient. Thus it would be a poor idea to perform amniocentesis at this time.

D. This patient has had no contractions, making tocolysis unnecessary at this time.

E. Betamethasone and dexamethasone have been shown to decrease rates of respiratory distress syndrome in neonates when given between 24 and 34 weeks of gestation. At this gestational age, the fetus is previable. Thus it is of little use to give antenatal corticosteroids at this point.

ANSWER 45

E. The patient has vulvovaginal candidiasis, which presents with pruritis, a white discharge, and may have an instigator such as a change in sexual habits, undergarments, or a course of antibiotics. Treatments for this include over-the-counter antifungal preparations (Monistat), prescription topical agents (Terazole cream), and oral fluconazole (Diflucan). The oral treatment is >85% effective from a one-time dose and is much more convenient than the topical agents.

A. Oral acyclovir would be used to treat or prophylax against herpes simplex virus (HSV) lesions.

B. Topical acyclovir is more often used for herpes labialis or herpetic lesions on the upper lip than herpes vaginalis or vulvar lesions.

C. Metronidazole can be used to treat bacterial vaginosis. Common dosing regimens include 500 mg PO BID and 250 mg PO TID.

D. Metronidazole can also be given in a vaginal preparation (Metro-gel).

ANSWER 46

D. There is a high association between cervical dysplasia, cervical cancer, and human papilloma virus (HPV). In particular, the subtypes that put one at risk include 16, 18, and 31, whereas subtypes 6 and 11 predispose to condyloma formation.

A. The average length of time to the development of cervical cancer with CIN I is 7 years, whereas CIN II can develop into carcinoma in 3–4 years. However, there are lesions that progress much faster. Thus, most patients are managed aggressively.

B. Thirty percent of CIN I lesions resolve spontaneously.

C & E. The next step in the management of a CIN I lesion would be scheduled colposcopy and directed biopsy. Colposcopy allows a better view of the cervix and uses acetic acid to bring out the possible lesions by turning them white. Once a formal diagnosis is made, CIN I lesions are usually followed every 3–4 months with colposcopy until the lesion either regresses or progresses. If a diagnosis is made at that time, cryotherapy or laser can be used. However, an excisional procedure that can demonstrate clear margins is often the procedure of choice with either the large loop excision of the transformation zone (LLETZ or LEEP) or a cold-knife-cone biopsy.

ANSWER 47

E. Infertility is defined as 12 months or more of unprotected intercourse not resulting in a pregnancy. It is estimated that 40% of infertility is male factor, 40% is female factor, and 20% is idiopathic (i.e., no etiology for the infertility is ever identified). Even in men who have conceived before, it is important to perform a semen analysis, particularly when the prior conception was many years ago. Chloride concentration is not routinely assessed in a semen analysis. However, dysfunctional chloride channels seen in patients with cystic fibrosis do lead to male factor infertility in most of those patients.

A. The semen analysis does include the ejaculatory volume, normally between 3 and 5 ml.

B. Sperm motility and morphology is also an important aspect of the semen analysis.

C. The pH of the semen is routinely checked.

D. The sperm and white blood cell concentration are routinely checked.

ANSWER 48

C. Tubal factor is thought to account for 30–40% of female factor infertility. The two primary tubal problems are occlusion and tubal dysfunction. Tubal occlusion can occur from pelvic adhesions from surgery, inflammation and/or infection, as well as purposely from a tubal ligation. Tubal dysfunction can result in the setting of endometriosis, internal tubal scarring from infection, Kartagener's syndrome, which causes abnormal cilial function, and smoking. There is little evidence to suggest that former use of an IUD in any way contributes to tubal occlusion or dysfunction. The rare case where this assertion might be made is when the patient had pelvic inflammatory disease in the setting of an IUD.

A. Pelvic inflammatory disease (PID) can cause scarring and adhesions that can lead to both extrinsic compression or occlusion of the tube as well as internal scarring and disruption in tubal motility.

B. While ectopic pregnancy may result from the same problems that can cause infertility, it is in itself associated with infertility, likely due to the treatment which can be either chemotherapy, which may lead to local scarring, or surgical.

D. Endometriosis, like PID, is felt to cause both occlusion and tubal dysfunction. One bit of evidence to support this is that patients with endometriosis and tubal patency have higher rates of infertility than the general population.

E. Both the local infection and inflammation secondary to appendicitis as well as the surgery itself can lead to pelvic adhesions that can cause tubal occlusion.

ANSWER 49

E. Endometrial cancer is the most common gynecologic cancer in the United States, affecting approximately 35,000 women annually. The median age of diagnosis is 61, with the majority of affected women in their 50s. It most commonly presents in postmenopausal women with vaginal bleeding or in premenopausal women with intermenstrual bleeding. It is commonly associated with unopposed estrogen. However, there is seemingly little increased risk in patients who take replacement estrogen with concomitant progesterone. Breast cancer patients who have been treated with tamoxifen are also at risk. Because estrogen exposure is a risk, nulliparity is also a risk factor for endometrial cancer.

A. Diabetes carries a relative risk of approximately 3 for endometrial cancer.

B. Hypertension is also associated with endometrial cancer.

C. Late menopause is associated with endometrial cancer, as are other physiologic states that result in long-term exposure to unopposed estrogen, such as anovulation.

D. Because peripheral conversion in adipose tissue increases estrogen levels, obesity is also a risk factor for endometrial cancer. Patients >50 lbs overweight carry a 10-fold increased risk over patients with normal weight.

ANSWER 50

A. This patient's history and physical are most consistent with stress incontinence, although a formal diagnosis is usually made with urodynamics. The fact that she leaks only with valsalva and physical activity is consistent with stress incontinence. Her risk factors include mild pelvic relaxation, childbirth, and the postmenopausal anestrogenic state. Her positive Q-tip test on physical exam further confirms the diagnosis. Stress incontinence can be treated medically with exercises, estrogen administration, and surgical restoration of the bladder neck to its original anatomic position.

B. Urge incontinence patients feel the urge to micturate and then urine begins to leak before they can get to the bathroom.

C. Detrusor instability is one etiology of urge incontinence. In addition, patients will occasionally have detrusor instability along with stress incontinence symptoms. Various stressors such as coughing can trigger detrusor contraction, leading to an appearance of stress incontinence that is actually detrusor instability. This can be diagnosed with urodynamics that reveal a detrusor contraction several seconds after a valsalva and leakage that occurs with the detrusor contraction rather than with the valsalva.

D. Total incontinence is rare and results from complete inability to maintain continence. It is most commonly seen in patients with fistulae from the bladder to the vagina or skin, or from the urethra or ureters to the vagina.

E. Overflow incontinence results from detrusor insufficiency or areflexia; that is, the bladder wall contracts weakly or not at all. In this case, urine collects in the bladder and dribbles out when the bladder capacity is exceeded.

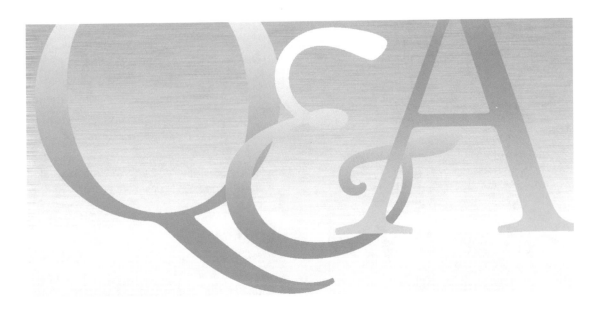

BLOCK **THREE**

ANSWERS

ANSWER 51

D. A low forceps delivery is defined as at least +2 station, meaning that the fetal skull is at least 2 cm below the ischial spines. It is broken up into rotations that are less than or more than 45°. An outlet forceps is when the fetal scalp is visible without separating the labia. A mid forceps is when the head is between 0 and +2 station and engaged. Anything above a mid forceps is a high forceps, which are no longer practiced in the United States because of association with fetal injury. In general, you should have the following in order to perform a delivery:

A. Adequate anesthesia, usually an epidural, but it can also be a pudendal or, rarely, a spinal.

B. See answer D.

C. A fetus that is not macrosomic. Macrosomia is associated with shoulder dystocia. Thus, it is not advisable to deliver the head only to cause a shoulder dystocia, which is associated with perinatal morbidity and mortality.

E. An obstetrician who is familiar with the indications and limitations of the use of obstetric forceps. Since the advent of the vacuum extractor, increasingly fewer obstetricians are trained in the use of forceps.

ANSWER 52

D. A first-degree relative with bilateral, premenopausal disease carries an 8-fold increase in breast cancer risk. This family history is the strongest risk factor in any patient, and management usually entails annual mammograms starting 10 years prior to when the relative was diagnosed with the disease.

A. Obesity carries a relative risk of 2.

B. Nulliparity is associated with a 3-fold risk of disease when compared to parous patients.

C. Hypertension appears associated with breast cancer, with an odds ratio between 1.2 and 1.5.

E. Diabetes, similar to hypertension, is weakly associated with breast cancer.

ANSWER 53

B. The average female patient has between 4 and 4.5 l of intravascular volume. Because this patient is larger than average, she may have as much as 5 l. Her blood loss during the case was approximately one-third of her total blood volume. In addition, she was given a large fluid bolus to replace the volume and now, 6 hr postoperatively, she has reequilibrated most of the fluids. Appropriately, her hematocrit is approximately two-thirds of her starting hematocrit.

A. In this stable patient with normal urine output, there is no reason to check serial hematocrits unless there was any concern that she may have continued intra-abdominal bleeding.

C. In this stable patient, there is no reason to reexplore.

D. With a hematocrit of 28 and a stable patient, there is no need to transfuse blood. Occasionally cancer patients or cardiac patients are transfused for hematocrits below 30 in order to prepare for chemotherapy or to maximize oxygen-carrying capacity.

E. There is no reason at this point to suspect a coagulopathy. If one was suspected, a better screening test is to check for fibrin split products such as the D-dimer.

ANSWER 54

A. Classically, to diagnose active phase arrest of labor or failure to progress in labor, adequate forces of labor must be demonstrated. The strength of contractions can be measured with an intrauterine pressure catheter (IUPC) since the external tocometer simply measures the frequency and duration of contractions. The units used most commonly to describe the forces of labor are Montevideo units. These are calculated by measuring the difference between the baseline and peak intrauterine pressures of the individual contractions summed over a 10-min period. Adequate forces are greater than or equal to 180–200 Montevideo units. Failure to progress in labor is usually defined when (1) adequate forces are demonstrated, and (2) the patient has no change in cervical dilation or station over a period of 2 hr in the active phase. At this point, cesarean delivery is commonly offered.

B. On the Friedman curve, a cervical dilation of at least 1 cm per hour is expected in the active phase, which is actually the 5th percentile of cervical change, i.e. 95% of all patients will dilate at 1 cm per hour or faster.

C. Commonly, if the forces of labor as measured are inadequate, oxytocin is begun and increased until contractions are considered adequate. Many patients will achieve adequate labor on their own and will not need oxytocin augmentation. Alternatively, if a patient is not making adequate progress, she is often begun on oxytocin augmentation prior to receiving the intrauterine pressure catheter.

D. Active phase arrest of labor is diagnosed when, in the setting of adequate forces of labor measured by an IUPC, there is no change in dilation or station during a 2-hr period.

E. The duration of active phase of labor differs between multiparous and nulliparous patients. The total length is not actually used to make the diagnosis of failure to progress. One reason for this is that a patient with inadequate labor may make slow cervical change for several hours before augmentation is begun, thus increasing the total length of labor.

ANSWER 55

D. Although most uterine perforations likely go unnoticed and most are not associated with morbidity or mortality, recognition of a uterine perforation requires that one evaluate the patient for stability and intra-abdominal bleeding. The least invasive way to do this is to perform a pelvic ultrasound to look for blood/fluid in the pelvis. In this case, because the hysteroscope had not begun, there should be minimal fluid in the pelvis.

A. If a uterine perforation is recognized, it is unsafe to proceed with hysteroscopy since the fluid under pressure is likely to pass in large amounts into the abdomen through the perforation site. In addition, placement of the hysteroscope may further dilate or damage the perforation site.

B. There is no need for laparotomy, unless there is evidence of intra-abdominal bleeding from the perforation site.

C. While laparoscopy could tell absolutely whether there is any ongoing bleeding from a perforation site, it is unnecessary in this case. The risks of performing a laparoscopy are not outweighed by the marginal increase in information gained over a pelvic ultrasound.

E. While it is true that most uterine perforations are not associated with long-term morbidity, it is still wise to admit the patient overnight for observation.

ANSWER 56

C. Fetal heart rate decelerations are generally a sign of acute decrease in oxygen, which leads to vagal stimulation and a decrease in the fetal heart rate. The decelerations described above are associated with contractions, begin after the contraction begins, and end after the contraction is over. This is a description of late decelerations, which are associated with uteroplacental insufficiency. Uteroplacental insufficiency itself can be caused by decreased maternal perfusion of the uterus secondary to anemia, hypoxia, or hypotension, as well as poor gas exchange across the placenta secondary to increased placental resistance or abruption.

A. Early decelerations begin and end with contractions and are thought to be due to fetal head compression.

B. Variable decelerations are not necessarily associated with contractions. They are sudden in onset, and the fetal heart rate reaches its nadir within 15–30 sec. These decelerations are thought to be secondary to umbilical cord compression.

D. Late decelerations are not caused by head compression.

E. A nuchal cord or umbilical cord that is wrapped around the fetal neck, is seen in 10–15% of pregnancies. As the fetus descends, the nuchal cord can be pulled and compressed, leading to variable decelerations.

ANSWER 57

D. Uterine atony is the most common etiology of postpartum hemorrhage. This patient has multiple risk factors for postpartum hemorrhage due to uterine atony, including chorioamnionitis, the use of magnesium sulfate, and a macrosomic fetus. In addition to uterine massage, uterine atony is treated with uterotonic agents such as oxytocin, prostaglandin F2alpha (Prostin), and methylergonovine (Methergine).

A. A cervical laceration is not an uncommon cause of a postpartum hemorrhage. This patient has one risk factor for cervical laceration, a macrosomic fetus. Other risk factors include a fast labor and pushing against a cervix that is not fully dilated. Cervical laceration is still much less likely than uterine atony.

B. A vaginal laceration, particularly one into the pelvic sidewall, can bleed quite impressively. Vaginal lacerations are more likely in the setting of an operative delivery.

C. While ruptured hemorrhoidal vessels are a common cause of bleeding postpartum, it is usually obvious when they are the etiology. The bleeding from this source is easily staunched during the repair of the perineum. However, in rare cases, hemorrhoidal vascular disruption can lead to hematomas and ongoing bleeding.

E. Retained products of conception such as a placental cotyledon or a succenturiate lobe may lead to uterine atony and postpartum hemorrhage. On examination, this patient's placenta was intact, and there was no evidence of a succenturiate lobe. In this setting, uterine exploration for retained products is indicated only after all other treatments have failed.

ANSWER 58

C. Ovarian cancer stage I is as follows: Ia is confined to one ovary, Ib is both ovaries, Ic is either a or b with rupture of the ovary, disease outside the capsule, or positive peritoneal washings.

A & B.   See C above

D & E.   See Table 58

Table 58   Staging of Ovarian Carcinoma

Stage II—Disease extends to the pelvis

a—Malignant cells in the uterus or fallopian tubes

b—Malignant cells elsewhere in the pelvis

c— a or b plus positive washings or disease beyond the capsule

Stage III—Disease extends to the abdomen

a—Only microscopic disease

b—Metastases <2 cm in size

c—Metastases >2 cm in size or any positive pelvic or para-aortic nodes

Stage IV—Distant metastases include positive pleural effusion and disease in the liver parenchyma.

ANSWER 59

D. Uric acid has been noted to be elevated in patients with preeclampsia, but has not been formally added to the diagnostic criteria or even the screening criteria. One study did show that it could be used to screen for preeclampsia among patients with renal disease and/or chronic hypertension who have normal baseline serum uric acid levels. In these high-risk patients, a uric acid that is increasing or that is higher than 6.0 is a good screening tool for preeclampsia.

A. Creatinine is essential to assess renal function. Creatinine in pregnancy should be low, certainly <0.7, because GFR is increased. A mildly elevated creatinine is often abnormal.

B. The CBC identifies the number of platelets, which is integral in screening for HELLP syndrome. The hematocrit can identify the degree of hemoconcentration.

C. The LFTs, particularly AST and ALT, need to be included in routine preeclamptic labs. Substantial elevation, particularly twice normal, is concerning.

E. LDH is a marker for hemolysis and should increase with HELLP syndrome, a variant of severe preeclampsia. Hemolysis can also be identified on a peripheral blood smear with evidence of schistocytes. However, the LDH is faster to obtain, and speed is important to the diagnosis of HELLP syndrome.

ANSWER 60

E. Twin pregnancies can be dizygotic (two initial zygotes) or monozygotic (one initial zygote that splits into two at some point). Dizygotic twins will always be dichorionic and diamnionic—two placentas and two amniotic cavities. Monozygotic twins can be di/di, mono/di, mono/mono, or conjoint (known by laypersons as Siamese), depending on when the zygote splits. At delivery, twin pregnancies can present in a variety of ways. Each fetus can be cephalic, breech, or transverse, creating nine possible presentations. If the presenting fetus is cephalic and the twins are concordant, a trial of labor with cephalic delivery or breech extraction of the second twin is reasonable.

A. Vaginal delivery of a breech presenting twin followed by a cephalic twin is usually not allowed. In addition to the usual risks of delivering the presenting twin breech, there is a risk of interlocking twins, where the second twin's head comes through the pelvis before the first twin's head.

B. After delivery of the first twin, the uterus rapidly decreases in size, which increases the risk for abruption of the second twin's placenta. Augmentation with high-dose Pitocin is likely to increase the risk of abruption and tetanic contractions. Classically, the occurrence of an undiagnosed twin is the reason Pitocin is not given until after delivery of the placenta.

C. Forceps should never be applied when the cervix is not fully dilated.

D. If both twins are cephalic presenting, there is no indication for cesarean delivery.

ANSWER 61

D. The patient's infertility in this case is most likely related to her endometriosis. However, with good tubal patency on the left and some spillage on the right, it is impossible to say for sure that tubal factor is implicated. Patients with infertility secondary to endometriosis will have increased fertility with the fulguration of implants that are seemingly unrelated to the adnexa.

A. With pelvic adhesions, chronic PID is in the differential. However with an endometrioma, endometriosis is the most likely diagnosis.

B. This is a possible etiology. However, with good tubal patency on the left it is impossible to make this diagnosis.

C. This patient with regular menses and documented ovulation does not have ovarian dysfunction.

E. This is incorrect on both accounts because there is a clear etiology, endometriosis, and tubal patency.

ANSWER 62

B. Heparin SQ dosed as 5000 BID or TID is most commonly used for DVT prophylaxis perioperatively. The original studies examined the TID dosing, which should be used in patients at highest risk, such as those with cancer. The BID dosing is commonly used in patients who are healthy and likely to mobilize quickly.

A. Coumadin has a slow onset and a long half-life. Thus, it is not used for perioperative prophylaxis.

C. LMW heparin such as Lovenox can be used for DVT prophylaxis, dosed at 40 units QD. However, because of its longer half-life than unfractionated heparin, it is not usually used perioperatively.

D & E. See Answers to A–C.

ANSWER 63

E. While it is often suggested to the patient that she should have adequate anesthesia, often via epidural, this is not an absolute contraindication to a vaginal breech delivery. Because of the likely need for piper forceps and possible need for emergent cesarean delivery, often patients undergoing a trial of labor for breech do receive epidural anesthesia.

A. Generally, the fetus undergoing breech delivery should be less than 4000 g, or not macrosomic. Some practitioners will use a lower cutoff of 3800 g because of the inaccuracy of ultrasound and Leopolds.

B. Breech fetuses can be in the frank, complete, or footling presentation. Fetuses in the footling breech presentation generally do not undergo a trial of labor because of the increased risk for cord prolapse.

C. Because the diameters of the head are minimized with flexion, the head of a breech fetus undergoing a trial of labor should be flexed in order to avoid head entrapment.

D. Most clinicians will not allow a fetus with anomalies to undergo a trial of labor in the breech position. The exception is a fetus that is not expected to live. In that setting, a trial of labor for a breech is preferable in order to avoid risks to the mother of cesarean delivery.

ANSWER 64

D. Erythromycin is used in conjunction with ampicillin in patients with preterm premature rupture of the membranes to promote prolonged latency period (time to delivery). However, erythromycin is not commonly used for prolonged latency or prophylaxis in patients with intact membranes.

A. Magnesium sulfate is commonly used for tocolysis in preterm labor. Other agents used for tocolysis include terbutaline, ritodrine, indomethacin, and nifedipine.

B. Penicillin is given to patients who are threatening to deliver preterm as prophylaxis against GBS.

C. Betamethasone is given to patients between 24 and 34 weeks GA at acute risk for preterm delivery in order to decrease the risk of respiratory distress syndrome and intraventricular hemorrhage.

E. GBS cultures are usually obtained in preterm patients. If they are negative, the penicillin can be stopped.

ANSWER 65

A. With a ureteral transection above the pelvic brim, the best repair is to reapproximate the two ends over a stent. The stent helps prevent stenosis from scarring during the healing process.

B. End-to-side reanastomosis is unusual in ureteral repair, and is used more in bowel reanastomosis to prevent stenotic sites.

C. If there is a distal ureteral injury, reimplantation may be used over reanastomosis. However, in this case the injury is too proximal to be reimplanted on the bladder.

D. An end-to-side anastomosis in ureteral repair may be used when implanting the ureter into the contralateral ureter. This is performed rarely in instances where the distal ureter has been resected and there is no way to gap the distance between the ureter and the bladder.

E. When the ureter has been damaged to such an extent that there is not enough distance to implant into the bladder or contralateral ureter, a nephrostomy tube that allows the kidney to continue functioning will be placed.

ANSWER 66

B. Currently, first-line combination chemotherapy for patients with epithelial ovarian carcinoma is Taxol and carboplatin. Carboplatin replaced cisplatin as the primary platinum-based alkylating agent because it is associated with fewer side effects.

A. CHOP is most commonly used for non-Hodgkin's lymphoma.

C. Melphalan was a commonly used single agent to treat ovarian cancer. It is still used in patients who are less likely to survive combination therapy because it is well tolerated.

D. Etoposide and cisplatin are most commonly used to treat oat cell lung cancer.

E. CMF combination chemotherapy has been used to treat breast cancer, with and without tamoxifen.

ANSWER 67

E. Expectant management for 96 hours is not a reasonable approach based upon evidence from a large randomized control trial in patients with term premature rupture of membranes (PROM). In that study, patients underwent expectant management for no longer than 72 hr. In the expectant management group, there was a slightly higher rate of maternal infection. In addition, these patients underwent fetal monitoring each day.

A & C. It is reasonable to begin induction immediately with no increase seen in either the rate of cesarean or the length of induction, whether induction is performed with prostaglandins or oxytocin.

B. There is some evidence from prospective studies that the rate of infection increases after 18 hr of rupture of membranes, so some clinicians will begin induction of labor 6–12 hr after rupture in order to maximize the chance that the patient delivers prior to the 18-hr threshold.

D. If expectant management at home is performed, it should last no more than 24 hr. In addition to daily fetal monitoring, the patient should check her temperature and return immediately for fever.

ANSWER 68

B. In the setting of an emergent cesarean delivery, it is reasonable to utilize spinal anesthesia as long as it can be administered quickly (<5 min) and there is no abruption, uterine rupture, or ongoing cause of severe hypoxia. In this case, given the reassuring fetal heart rate, spinal anesthesia is preferred as the head is lifted off of the cord.

A. Epidural anesthesia takes longer to achieve a surgical level, and is less often successful than spinal anesthesia. Epidural anesthesia is excellent for labor because continuous administration and titration for less neuromuscular block are possible.

C. In a true emergent cesarean delivery, if the anesthesiologist does not normally place many spinals, general anesthesia is commonly used. This patient may not be a good candidate for intubation, given her history of scleroderma. Hopefully, the patient and her airway were evaluated by anesthesia at admission.

D. Occasionally, if anesthesia is unavailable, a cesarean section will be performed under local anesthesia with conscious sedation. This is certainly not an optimal way to perform surgery, and given the presence of an obstetric anesthesiologist in this case, is unnecessary.

E. Pudendal anesthesia may be administered by an obstetrician prior to performing an operative vaginal delivery with vacuum or forceps.

ANSWER 69

E. Laparoscopic injuries to the bowel are rare and dangerous complications. The bowel can be injured during insertion of the Veress needle, insertion of the trochars, operative dissection, using sharp instruments and use of electrocautery—particularly unipolar electrocautery that can lead to arcing of sparks. Patients can present immediately or several days post-op with symptoms related to bowel perforation. In this patient with an acute abdomen and septic physiology, a bowel injury leading to a perforation is the most likely diagnosis. Of note, a KUB and upright are of little use since the patient will have free air in her abdomen from the surgery.

A. Post-op PID is unlikely in this patient, and is usually seen in patients after the release of a hydrosalpinx that is filled with contaminated material. Her signs and symptoms indicate a systemic problem, and are more consistent with the rupture of a viscus.

B. Endomyometritis should not create such widespread abdominal symptoms.

C. Appendicitis can present like this, but given the timing of the recent surgery, bowel injury is more likely. In either situation, consultation with general surgery and immediate abdominal exploration is the next step.

D. It is unlikely that ureteral injury would present with signs of infection and subsequent progression to sepsis.

ANSWER 70

E. The most common cause of ambiguous genitalia is congenital adrenal hyperplasia (CAH). Three common enzyme deficiencies can lead to CAH: (1) 3-beta-hydroxy-steroid dehydrogenase; (2) 11-beta-hydroxylase; and most commonly (3) 21-hydroxylase. The last, 21-hydroxylase deficiency, leads to accumulation of 17-hydroxyprogesterone and a deficiency of cortisol and the mineralocorticoids. Testosterone is slightly elevated, and progesterone and estrogen are usually normal. Thus, male fetuses usually have entirely normal appearance, but female newborns may have ambiguous genitalia. Medical treatment involves replacement of the missing steroid hormones.

A. Corrective surgery should be deferred for at least several months to allow for adjustment to medical therapy, but should be performed before the child can remember the gender confusion. Parents may push to have the surgery as soon as possible.

B. Estradiol is usually normal.

C. Progesterone will be either normal or slightly elevated, and does not need replacement.

D. Testosterone is likely elevated in this newborn, leading to the ambiguous genitalia.

ANSWER 71

B. While variable decelerations and even prolonged decelerations are a relatively common phenomenon during labor, the sudden change of the fetal station from +2 to unpalpable and high is abnormal and highly concerning. In this setting of a patient undergoing a trial of labor having had a prior cesarean delivery, the most likely diagnosis is a uterine rupture. Other common signs and symptoms associated with uterine rupture include a maternal "popping" sensation in the abdomen, extreme abdominal pain, palpation of fetal parts outside the uterus, gush of vaginal bleeding, and maternal hypotension secondary to intra-abdominal bleeding. Even with the fetal heart rate improving, a rapid cesarean delivery is indicated.

A. This would be a reasonable next step if the fetal head was palpable.

C. Forceps cannot be used with a fetal head this high or a cervix that is not fully dilated.

D. Expectant management would be reasonable if uterine rupture did not appear to be the likely diagnosis. If the head were still at +2 station and there were no recurrences of the prolonged decelerations, the patient would hopefully be completely dilated soon and could be delivered vaginally.

E. As with expectant management, if you did not suspect uterine rupture, you would restart the Pitocin about 20–30 min after the prolonged deceleration.

ANSWER 72

D. With presumed pelvic inflammatory disease (PID) and no resolution of symptoms or signs after 48 hr of appropriate treatment, the patient is at risk for a tubo-ovarian abscess (TOA). This is best diagnosed by pelvic ultrasound. Furthermore, given her symptoms, pelvic ultrasound should probably have been performed on admission to rule out TOA.

A. Laparoscopy is used in some facilities to diagnose PID, but would be of little use at this point in this patient.

B. If the patient has a TOA that does not respond to more aggressive antibiotics, she may require surgical treatment. Because she is a young woman, and surgical management often involves salpingo-oophorectomy, conservative management with antibiotics is usually first-line therapy.

C. Cultures from the cervix can be useful to fine-tune antibiotic treatment. In this patient who is not responding to medical therapy, broadening treatment is likely to be more effective than waiting for culture results.

E. While broadening coverage may be necessary, ampicillin and gentamicin would need to be given with clindamycin for coverage of chlamydia and anaerobic organisms.

ANSWER 73

D. In this patient with gestational diabetes and a history of a macrosomic birth, you should be prepared for the possibility of a shoulder dystocia. This includes alerting the nursing staff of your suspicion, having extra help in the room, flexing the patient's thighs for delivery, and having someone ready to apply suprapubic pressure after delivery of the head, if necessary.

A. A forceps delivery is unnecessary in this case. Further, given your suspicion for macrosomia, the use of forceps or vacuum to perform an operative vaginal delivery is inadvisable.

B. See answer A.

C. A cesarean delivery is unnecessary at this point, with vaginal delivery being imminent. Rarely, if a severe shoulder dystocia cannot be resolved after 5–6 min of maneuvers, the fetal head is pushed back into the maternal pelvis and a cesarean delivery is performed. This is called a Zavanelli maneuver and is the procedure of last resort in a shoulder dystocia.

E. Uterine inversion is more common in multiparous women and with macrosomic fetuses. It is uncommon, and unlikely to occur in this patient.

ANSWER 74

C. Wound infections are the most common complication of abdominal and pelvic surgery. They can be a simple cellulitis, wound abscess, or a fasciitis, which carries with it a relatively high rate of mortality. The next step in this patient's management is to further assess the wound. The simplest way to do this is at the bedside with local anesthesia. The incision should then be opened 1–2 cm to allow for exploration of the wound with a cotton swab. If the abscess is local and without much depth, the wound can be irrigated and packed with cotton gauze.

A. The patient may require intravenous antibiotics, depending on the extent of the wound infection. If the patient is admitted with a fasciitis, broad spectrum antibiotics should be given. However, with a small wound abscess that is opened and packed, continuing the oral antibiotics for the accompanying cellulitis should be adequate.

B. If the infection is found to be quite extensive, or if the patient does not tolerate examination under local anesthesia, exploration in the OR may be necessary.

D. The wound should be irrigated, but not until it is explored.

E. A CT scan is sometimes used if a wound is closed and without obvious fluctuence or if the cellulitis does not resolve after treatment. The CT can identify any enclosed areas of fluid or an intra-abdominal abscess.

ANSWER 75

A. This patient is likely intravascularly depleted. The first step in dealing with her oliguria is to give IV fluid. Patients who undergo abdominal surgery have large insensible losses. This patient also had approximately 4 l of ascites drained, is likely quite dry, and should receive aggressive rehydration. Of note, overly aggressive rehydration can cause pulmonary edema.

B. While this patient is likely down several liters of total fluid, a 2000 cc bolus is a bit aggressive in this situation.

C. Salt poor albumin (SPA) may be useful for this patient if several boluses of crystalloid have failed to result in adequate urination. Patients with ovarian cancer often have low oncotic pressure secondary to low albumin, and boluses of colloid can improve intravascular volume at least temporarily.

D & E. Only if the patient normally takes a diuretic should one be given in the first 24 hr post-op for oliguria. While there is likely to be a response, the diuretic may leave the patient with even less intravascular fluid and may increase the risk of acute renal failure.

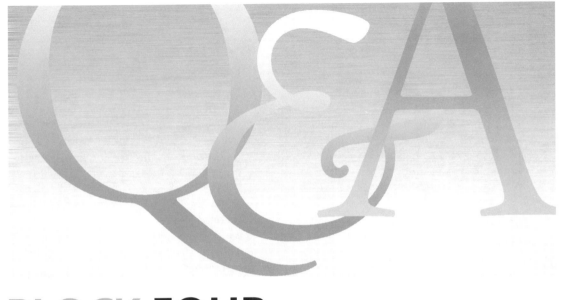

BLOCK FOUR

ANSWERS

ANSWER 76

E. It is important to continue breast-feeding or pumping breast milk during the acute phase of the infection in order to prevent the intraductal accumulation of infected material. Patients should be reassured that since most cases of mastitis are caused by the patient's skin flora or the infant's oral flora, it is not harmful to continue breast-feeding.

A. Breast pain due to mastitis can be treated symptomatically with NSAIDs.

B & C. Mastitis can be treated by oral antibiotics that will cover maternal skin flora or the infant's oral flora. Commonly prescribed agents are dicloxacillin or Keflex for 7–10 days.

D. Application of warm compresses to the affected breast will increase blood flow to the affected area and expedite healing.

ANSWER 77

C. Adnexal torsion is the twisting of the ovary or adnexa about the ovarian pedicle, resulting in vascular obstruction. Although uncommon, it is an emergency and requires operative intervention. Patients occasionally report prior occurrences of similar pain as the offending cyst or neoplasm enlarges. It is associated with a normal temperature and white count, nausea, and vomiting. Diagnosis can be confirmed by ultrasound, which typically shows an enlarged ovary that may contain a cyst or be uniformly echogenic with decreased Doppler flow. Figure 77 shows absent drastolic flow and an enlarged ovary with a simple cyst.

A. Although this patient has pain localizing to the RLQ, acute appendicitis generally presents with anorexia, fever, leukocytosis, and not uncommonly, an acute abdomen. With an identifiable adnexal mass, the etiology of the pain is unlikely to be due to other causes.

B. The patient has a negative pregnancy test. Additionally, an early ectopic pregnancy is unlikely to produce such symptoms.

D. Salpingitis typically presents with fever, elevated white count, vaginal discharge, and cervical motion tenderness.

E. Although certainly more common than adnexal torsion, ruptured ovarian cysts typically produce pain that is bilateral and begins at or after ovulation. Were this truly rupture of an ovarian cyst, there is usually more diffuse pelvic pain and peritoneal signs. Also, the patient might have presented with a decreased hematocrit if bleeding were severe. Ultrasound would show free fluid in the cul-de-sac and is less likely than torsion to reveal the presence of an enlarged adnexal mass.

ANSWER 78

D. In an inevitable abortion, there will be vaginal bleeding and a dilated cervix but no expulsion of products of conception. Although the use of prostaglandins to promote the expulsion of the products of conception is an option, dilatation and curettage is preferential in the setting of heavy bleeding. Of note, if this patient were Rh D (–), Rhogam administration would be necessary to prevent alloimmunization in subsequent pregnancies. Figure 78 shows a large, empty intrauterine gestational sac. A gestational sac this size should have a fetal pole.

A. Any pregnant woman presenting with vaginal bleeding and abdominal pain must be ruled out for ectopic pregnancy. The presence of an intrauterine gestational sac makes the likelihood of a concurrent extrauterine pregnancy highly unlikely, but ectopic pregnancy must still be excluded by history, physical examination, labs, and a careful survey of the lower pelvis by ultrasound.

B. A threatened abortion is defined by vaginal bleeding in a viable pregnancy in the presence of a closed cervical os and no expulsion of products of conception. In the setting of a desired pregnancy, the patient should be given instructions for pelvic rest and followed for continued bleeding rather than proceed prematurely to definitive procedures such as dilatation and curettage.

C. An incomplete abortion is the partial expulsion of products of conception prior to 20 weeks gestation. It can either be allowed to complete on its own, or the patient can be offered dilatation and curettage or dilatation and evacuation.

E. A complete abortion is the complete expulsion of all products of conception prior to 20 weeks gestation. Patients should be followed for signs of infection and recurrent bleeding.

ANSWER 79

B. Approximately 20% of vaginal bleeding in postmenopausal women is due to cancer. In particular, endometrial cancer is the most common gynecologic malignancy in the USA, causing 50–60% of postmenopausal bleeding in women greater than 80 years. Endometrial biopsy is the gold standard for diagnosing endometrial cancer because of the ease with which it can be performed. However, if this patient were experiencing heavy, ongoing bleeding, a D & C would be more appropriate as it would both stop the bleeding and obtain a specimen for pathology.

A. Cervical etiologies are unlikely in a woman with a recently normal Pap smear and no visible lesion or history of trauma. It is still necessary to rule out cervical cancer as an etiology for bleeding, but the incidence of endometrial cancer is higher and should therefore be investigated first.

C. Although hysteroscopy would be useful in identifying potential causes for bleeding, such as endometrial polyps and myomas, malignant etiologies should be addressed first. Given the thickened endometrium (>5 mm in postmenopausal women) found on ultrasound, the endometrium should be assessed prior to proceeding with hysteroscopy.

D. See answer B.

E. Given the high likelihood of malignancy, attempting to manage the bleeding medically without first evaluating potential etiologies is inappropriate.

ANSWER 80

A. Mittelschmerz (from German—literally "middle pain") is pain due to the rupture of an ovarian follicle during ovulation resulting in intraperitoneal fluid or blood that can produce localized or diffuse abdominal pain. The easiest way to prevent future bouts of mittelschmerz is to place the patient on OCPs to suppress ovulation.

B. PID is most commonly seen in young, sexually active women with multiple partners. In addition to being in a long-term monogamous relationship, this patient is unlikely to have PID because she is afebrile, has a normal white count, and no cervical motion tenderness or vaginal discharge.

C. Patients with mittelschmerz can be confused with adnexal torsion frequently. The timing and nature of the symptoms in this patient make mittelschmerz a more likely diagnosis. One would expect a more protracted course in adnexal torsion, usually with concomitant nausea and vomiting. A pelvic ultrasound may help in the differential in a more confusing picture.

D. The patient has a negative pregnancy test.

E. Left-sided pain can occur uncommonly in acute appendicitis. However, the patient does not have other signs or symptoms that are consistent with appendicitis.

ANSWER 81

C. Because untreated PID can lead to infertility, hospitalization is generally recommended for reproductive-aged patients. However, it is highly recommended that adolescents or any patient in whom compliance may be an issue be hospitalized for treatment.

A. Both maternal and fetal consequences of PID exist that necessitate hospitalization. Gonococcal infection has been strongly linked to septic spontaneous abortion. Chlamydial infection can lead to neonatal conjunctivitis and pneumonias.

B. Severely ill patients not tolerating oral intake are unlikely to comply with medication regimens and will need hospitalization for parenteral therapy.

D. If a patient who is undergoing outpatient management of PID presents with worsening symptoms, becomes unable to tolerate POs, or has an unresolving physical exam on follow-up exam, she should be admitted for parenteral therapy.

E. See answer C.

ANSWER 82

A. Emergency contraception is effective up to 72 hr after the act of unprotected intercourse. The most common regimen is to use two pills of 50 μg of ethinyl estradiol and 0.5 mg of norgestrel (Ovral), given 12 hr apart for a total of four pills. It is currently available in combination with a urine pregnancy test.

B. Although the data is insufficient to evaluate the teratogenic risk to the pregnancy, it is still prudent to rule out the presence of a preexisting pregnancy.

C. Nausea occurs in 30–66% of patients receiving emergency oral contraception.

D. Ninety-eight percent of patients will menstruate by 21 days after the treatment.

E. Multiple agents exist for emergency contraception, but emergency contraception using oral contraceptives is prescribed most often.

ANSWER 83

E. This patient has a ruptured ectopic pregnancy based on the fact that she has no identifiable intrauterine pregnancy at a gestational age where one should easily be found by ultrasound. Additionally, she has free fluid in the cul-de-sac and a history of PID, which is a known risk factor for ectopic pregnancy. The decision to take the patient emergently to the operating room is based on the high probability for a ruptured ectopic pregnancy that is likely to have ongoing bleeding.

A. Unnecessary, as the diagnosis is highly likely, given the ultrasound findings.

B. See answer A.

C & D. Although serial quantitative βhCG levels would have been helpful in diagnosis prior to rupture, obtaining a value now does not affect management. Medical management is not indicated once the ectopic pregnancy has ruptured.

ANSWER 84

D. Despite no initial visual evidence of sperm on a wet prep slide, it is still possible that intravaginal ejaculation did occur. Thus, she should be offered emergency contraception. A baseline pregnancy test is also performed, and if she does not have menses within 21 days, she is advised to see her gynecologist for follow up.

A. This is the most common form of emergency contraception used.

B. Azithromycin 1 g PO covers *Chlamydia trachomatis* and Ceftriaxone 250 mg IM covers *Neisseria gonorrhoeae*.

C. Even if she objects to having this crime reported, it is a reportable crime. Often, the nursing staff in the ED will already have done so, but it is important that the physician seeing the patient follows up and makes sure the crime has been reported. Along these lines, evidence of the crime needs to be collected as well. The patient can then decide not to give a report to the police once they are involved.

E. If the patient was exposed to HIV, she will not show any evidence yet. However, it is important to obtain baseline testing.

ANSWER 85

B. This patient has a presentation that is worrisome for toxic shock syndrome (TSS). There is no data to support an association between PCOS and TSS. The other potential causes provide portals of entry for infection. One of the most commonly associated findings with TSS is a highly absorbent tampon.

A. The *Staphylococcus aureus* toxic shock syndrome toxin-1 has been implicated in TSS. Its systemic absorption leads to fever, rash, and desquamation of palms and soles.

C. Because the exotoxin is absorbed through the vaginal wall, blood cultures are usually negative.

D. TSS carries a high mortality rate, and thus all patients should be hospitalized. In severe cases, pressors may be required to stabilize blood pressures. With aggressive supportive management, it is likely that mortality can be reduced.

E. There have been less than 300 cases of TSS reported per year since 1984.

ANSWER 86

B. Although the fetal heart rate (FHR) tracing is concerning because it is nonreactive, there is no evidence of acute fetal insult (FHR decelerations or absent variability) that would necessitate emergent delivery at this time. Attempts should be made to achieve a reactive tracing by VAS, fetal scalp stimulation (difficult in this patient with a high cervix) or to obtain a biophysical profile (BPP).

A. Although elevated, the patient's glucose level does not warrant additional insulin at this time. There is no reason to react to a blood sugar less than 200 in this setting.

C. Assuming the gestational age is accurate, there is no evidence of fetal benefit from administration of betamethasone beyond 34 weeks of gestation.

D & E. Delivery is not indicated in this patient unless the FHR tracing becomes nonreassuring. If that were the case, the decision regarding route of delivery would depend on the severity of the nonreassuring FHR tracing as well as fetal presentation. If induction of labor were indicated rather than emergent cesarean section, a prostaglandin agent would be appropriate in this patient with an unfavorable cervix.

ANSWER 87

D. Because of her history of manual placenta extraction, this patient is at increased risk for development of endomyometritis, which is a polymicrobial infection of the uterine lining and wall. Diagnosis is made by the presence of fever, uterine tenderness, and elevated white count. Treatment is with broad-spectrum antibiotics. Dilation and curettage is only indicated if retained products of conception is suspected, which is not the case in this patient whose lochia has decreased appropriately.

A. Given her history of decreased vaginal bleeding, stable vital signs and hematocrit, this patient does not have a delayed postpartum hemorrhage.

B. Placenta accreta (abnormal adherence of the placenta to the uterine wall) would manifest as continued vaginal bleeding unresponsive to contractile agents and is more likely to be diagnosed immediately postpartum rather than 1 week later.

C. The patient has no evidence of a vaginal hematoma, which occurs when the trauma of delivery injures a blood vessel without disrupting the overlying epithelium. Vaginal hematomas commonly manifest as back pain and a large drop in the hematocrit. They can be managed expectantly, unless the patient is hemodynamically unstable, in which case surgical exploration and ligation of the disrupted vessel(s) may be required.

E. See answer D.

ANSWER 88

B. A lesion that is confined to the cervix, >5 mm invasive, and <4 cm wide is a Stage Ib1 lesion. Approximately 40% of cervical cancer is Stage Ib at diagnosis, which has an 85% cure rate regardless of whether radical hysterectomy or radiation therapy is used. For bulky Stage Ib to IVa disease, primary treatment with cisplatin-based chemotherapy in conjunction with radiation therapy can prolong disease-free survival when compared to radiation therapy alone.

A. This is Stage Ib1 disease; cone biopsy is only appropriate in microinvasive disease (Stage Ia1 and Ia2).

C. Stage Ib2 lesions are > 4 cm wide.

D & E. Stage II lesions extend beyond the cervix but not to the sidewall, with vaginal involvement in the upper 2/3 only. IIa lesions do not involve the parametria whereas IIb lesions have obvious parametrial involvement. Radical hysterectomy is only beneficial treatment for Stage IIa disease or less. Radiation therapy is indicated once the cancer has spread to the parametria or beyond (Stage IIb or greater). As above, primary chemotherapy can be beneficial for both IIa and IIb disease.

See Table 88

Table 88   Staging Cervical Cancer

Stage I—Confined to the cervix
    IA—Microscopic Disease
    IB—Clinically identifiable lesions

Stage II—Extracervical, but not to the pelvic walls or distal third of the vagina
    IIA—No parametrial involvement
    IIB—Parametrial involvement

Stage III—Extension to the pelvic wall or distal vagina
    IIIA—Not to the pelvic wall
    IIIB—To the pelvic wall

Stage IV—Beyond the true pelvis
    IVA—To the bladder or rectum
    IVB—Distant metastases

ANSWER 89

E. This patient is most likely having a placental abruption secondary to her elevated blood pressures and possible preeclampsia. Although the patient is hemodynamically stable and the fetus is premature, emergent delivery by cesarean section is indicated because of nonreassuring fetal status. It is reasonable to check the fetal heart rate in the OR to verify that it is still decreased; this will help further guide the rapidity with which the delivery needs to occur.

A. The patient may require blood transfusion because the volume of blood loss in a placental abruption is often underestimated due to concealed bleeding. However, this is not the most appropriate next step given the nonreassuring FHR tracing.

B. Although the fetus is premature and would likely benefit from the administration of betamethasone, immediate delivery is indicated, and thus there would not be sufficient time to benefit from corticosteroid effects.

C. The use of tocolytics to prolong the pregnancy until fetal lung maturity can be achieved might be indicated in a stable abruption, which is not the case here. If the patient is having a tetanic contraction, it is reasonable to give terbutaline, 0.25 mg SQ to promote uterine relaxation.

D. Induction of labor is inappropriate since emergent delivery is indicated.

ANSWER 90

E. All of the above are appropriate options in the management of pulmonary embolus in postpartum patients.

A. True, but it should not be the only treatment administered to the patient, as she will also require medical therapy.

B. This is often the initial medical therapy of choice. Conversion to subcutaneous heparin can occur after 10 days of IV heparin. If conversion to warfarin is desired, both IV heparin and warfarin should be administered for the first 5–7 days to ensure proper conversion. Warfarin is not utilized during pregnancy due to concern regarding teratogenicity. Although the American Academy of Pediatrics considers warfarin to be compatible with breast-feeding, concerned mothers can choose to convert to subcutaneous heparin instead of warfarin.

C. Treating an acute DVT or PE is now often accomplished with low molecular weight heparin. This allows patients to be discharged as soon as they are stable.

D. See answer B.

ANSWER 91

E. By her history and physical, the patient has a small bowel obstruction (SBO). Her KUB and upright confirm this and are further worrisome for bowel perforation with evidence of free air. This patient needs IVs placed for rehydration and immediate exploration in the OR. She should be consented for possible bowel resection, possible ileostomy, and/or colostomy.

A. In patients with SBO who are stable, NGT placement and NPO are reasonable plans for management.

B. Although this patient may require TPN at a later time, she has a SBO that has likely perforated and requires emergent laparotomy prior to management of her malnutrition.

C. Laparoscopy is now being utilized for second-look operations for confirmation of absent disease in ovarian cancer. However, it is not the issue in this patient.

D. In a patient with appendicitis or cholecystitis, this approach is sometimes taken. However, in this patient who has a perforated viscous, she needs to go to the OR immediately.

ANSWER 92

B. Since continuous OCPs have proven to be effective for this patient, she should be restarted on them. The patient should be informed that she can withdraw from the OCPs approximately twice a year and that it is acceptable to not have regular menses given the cyclical nature of endometriosis pain.

A. This regimen has proven to be ineffective for the patient in the past and there is no reason to believe that resuming it now would provide pain relief for the patient.

C. Although menstrual suppression by progestin treatment, usually medroxyprogesterone depot injection, is effective treatment for some women with endometriosis, it is preferable to resume an effective treatment rather than experiment with new regimens.

D. GnRH agonists are effective in treating chronic endometriosis pain in 75–90% of women. However, their use is generally limited to 6 months due to the side effects associated with estrogen deficiency (bone loss and vasomotor symptoms). Although "add-back" regimens have been utilized successfully to counter these side effects, this is tempered by the inconvenience and cost of additional medication. Additionally, the long-term effects of extended (>6 months) GnRH treatment have not been assessed. As mentioned in the prior answer choice, it is preferable to resume an effective treatment rather than experiment with new regimens.

E. There is no indication for operative treatment in this patient with endometriosis responsive to medical treatment and no desire for future fertility.

ANSWER 93

D. The goals of management in patients with severe hyperemesis gravidarum include maintenance of hydration and nutritional status, as well as symptom relief. Achievement of these goals requires a team approach and often includes consultation of social work and nutrition services. Although many patients will respond to IV hydration and antiemetics, a small percentage of patients may require prolonged hospitalization. If, in this setting, POs cannot be tolerated, it is then reasonable to place a pediatric feeding tube, which is usually well tolerated. Only after attempting every other form of nutrition and hydration should TPN be considered.

A. Hospitalization will be required if the patient cannot tolerate POs.

B. Many patients with hyperemesis gravidarum are conflicted about the pregnancy, and a social services consult can provide the added social support they may need.

C. Zofran has been used in pregnancy in these patients for several years with no known teratogenic effects. It is commonly reserved for nausea and vomiting refractory to other first-line antiemetic agents.

E. If the patient cannot take POs, a feeding tube should be placed. The feeding tube's tip is in the duodenum, thus the feeds are usually tolerated very well. This is the preferred method feeding as compared to TPN.

ANSWER 94

A. Although numerous risk factors exist for preterm delivery, the biggest risk factor is history of a prior preterm delivery. Other risk factors for preterm labor include multiple gestations, polyhydramnios, African American race, bacterial vaginosis, uterine anomalies, preterm rupture of the membranes, preeclampsia, and some maternal medical conditions.

B. While it has been theorized that multiple TABs increase the risk of incompetent cervix, there have been no studies to date that correlate history of one prior TAB with preterm delivery.

C. Bacterial vaginosis has been associated with preterm labor, but no such association exists with vaginal candidiasis.

D. A prepregnancy weight of <50 kg is a risk factor for preterm delivery, but no such association exists with obesity.

E. While it is true that maternal age <20 is associated with preterm delivery, this is not the patient's biggest risk factor.

ANSWER 95

E. The patient is experiencing dysmenorrhea secondary to outflow obstruction. She has cervical stenosis, which is a known complication of LEEP and other cervical surgeries. The most appropriate treatment for this patient is cervical dilatation, as oral contraceptives will only decrease the amount of her menstrual flow but not actually resolve the underlying problem. Unfortunately, many patients with cervical stenosis will experience recurrences of the disorder, requiring repeat cervical dilations.

A. Although the patient has a history of instrumentation, she does not have any evidence of infection, making pelvic abscess an unlikely etiology for her symptoms.

B. Although dysmenorrhea is a common symptom of endometriosis, the rest of the patient's history is inconsistent with such a diagnosis, which can only be truly made by diagnostic laparoscopy.

C. It is highly unlikely that the patient would develop cervical cancer after being diagnosed with cervical dysplasia and undergoing LEEP only 6 months ago. Additionally, cervical cancer often presents as painless postcoital vaginal bleeding rather than dysmenorrhea.

D. See answer E.

ANSWER 96

B. This patient has a mild case of ovarian hyperstimulation syndrome (OHSS), a rare but potentially life-threatening complication of ovulation induction with gonadotropins. In addition to ovarian enlargement, these patients also experience weight gain and abdominal distention. In severe cases, patients can present with ascites, pleural effusion, electrolyte imbalance, hypovolemia, and oliguria. The syndrome is managed by hospitalization, discontinuing gonadotropins, correcting fluid and electrolyte imbalances, and supportive therapy as needed.

A. While adnexal torsion is relatively common in OHSS, the patient's exam and history are not consistent with such a diagnosis. For a diagnosis of adnexal torsion, one would expect nausea, vomiting, and a more concerning pelvic exam.

C. Ectopic pregnancy should be considered in the differential diagnosis of any sexually active woman of childbearing age who presents with lower abdominal pain. However, the negative pregnancy test and large ovarian mass on ultrasound examination make such a diagnosis unlikely. Because the possibility of an early ectopic pregnancy exists, a quantitative beta-hCG would assist in confirming the diagnosis.

D. While the patient may have an endometrioma in the pelvis, her acute symptoms are more consistent with OHSS.

E. The patient's history of an occluded left fallopian tube might make the diagnosis of PID more likely. However, with the exception of abdominal pain, she has no physical signs or symptoms of PID.

ANSWER 97

A. Complete moles result from the fertilization of an empty ovum by a normal sperm, which is then thought to duplicate itself. Thus, the most common karyotype for complete moles is 46, XX. A partial mole is the fertilization of an ovum with two sperm, and the most common karyotype is 69, XXY.

B–D. Treatment of complete moles is with immediate suction evacuation of the uterus and gentle curettage. They cannot be managed expectantly, and a hysterectomy would be too extreme. Chemotherapy is only indicated if malignant transformation occurs, which is confirmed by persistently elevated beta-hCG levels after uterine evacuation.

E. The risk of developing GTD in subsequent pregnancies is only 5%.

ANSWER 98

D. The patient is experiencing urinary retention. Given her recent history of urogynecological surgery, the likely etiology is overcorrection of her urinary incontinence with resultant urinary outflow obstruction. The appropriate treatment is placement of a Foley catheter to relieve the obstruction. Surgical exploration and repair are not indicated at this time.

A–C. Although the patient's urine sample was not an ideal specimen, the lack of leukocyte esterase on urine dipstick makes the diagnosis of UTI unlikely. If clinical suspicion for infection is high, the urine should be cultured. A straight catheter specimen is not necessary and a single catheterization will not correct this patient's problem. However, once the Foley catheter is placed, antibiotic suppression against UTIs is usually started.

E. The patient may eventually need a repeat surgery to relax the suspension of the bladder neck. However, this should not happen immediately, nor without another trial of voiding.

ANSWER 99

D. Magnesium sulfate has been shown to be the most effective agent in preventing recurrent seizures in eclamptic patients. Magnesium sulfate can also be effective in interrupting the event, and can usually be given as a 10 g IM load to patients without an IV placed.

A. Until recently, phenytoin remained the drug of choice to prevent recurrent seizures in eclampsia in much of the world. However, there have been several studies that have demonstrated magnesium sulfate's efficacy.

B. If the patient were still actively seizing, diazepam or another short-acting benzodiazepine could be used to break the ongoing seizure activity.

C. Like phenytoin, phenobarbital may help prevent recurrent seizures, but does not seem to be as effective in randomized trials.

E. Expectant management is not appropriate. The patient needs active seizure prophylaxis and should be delivered unless severely remote from term.

ANSWER 100

B. Cyclic OCPs are the best treatment option for this patient with menorrhagia and dysmenorrhea. Over a period of 6 months, her symptoms should diminish and eventually, women who cycle on OCs will have minimal bleeding because of the endometrial atrophy that develops on OCs.

A. In the absence of ongoing vaginal bleeding (soaking >1 pad/hour), D&C is not indicated.

C & E. Neither GnRH nor progestin therapy are appropriate treatment options for this patient.

D. Although endometrial ablation would likely stop the patient's bleeding, it would also compromise her future fertility and is therefore not the best treatment option.